Paul Robinson
Sept 04

Complexity for Clinicians

Edited by
Tim A Holt
Clinical Lecturer
Centre for Primary Health Care Studies
University of Warwick

Foreword by
Marshall Marinker

Radcliffe Publishing
Oxford • San Francisco

Radcliffe Publishing Ltd
18 Marcham Road
Abingdon
Oxon OX14 1AA
United Kingdom

www.radcliffe-oxford.com
Electronic catalogue and worldwide online ordering.

British Library Cataloguing in Publication Data

A catalogue record for this book is available from the British Library.

ISBN 1 85775 855 2

Typeset by Aarontype Ltd, Easton, Bristol
Printed and bound by TJ International Ltd, Padstow, Cornwall

Contents

Foreword

The clinician's training in diagnostic reasoning implies, indeed requires, the existence of robust linear relationships – for example between epidemiological data and the risks and incidence of disease; between clinical findings and their underlying causes; between diagnosis and treatment. Yet, although generally reliable, these relationships become less than securely embedded in the evidence at the very point where the doctor has most need of them – in addressing the unique patient and her particular predicament. This is not because the data are inherently flawed or incomplete, but because they are derived from the study of large populations. What can be claimed to be generally 'true' for such researched populations cannot simultaneously be true for each of the individual patients included in them. Confronted by the actual patient, our linear rationality, based on such evidence from populations, begins to falter.

Some years ago I suggested the following division of diagnostic labour. The diagnostic task of the specialist is to limit uncertainty, to explore possibility and to marginalise error. That of the generalist is to tolerate uncertainty, to explore probability and to marginalise danger. Yet all clinicians, whatever their degree of subspecialisation, have to manage an irreducible uncertainty.

What do we mean by this uncertainty? It is not the consequence of ignorance of facts or failure of logic. It is rather the inevitable consequence of all those givens addressed by 'complexity' – the multiplicity, the multi-level, diverse, interconnectedness and dynamism, of events.

For example, as we contemplate the impact of genomics on clinical science and practice, we are struck by the astronomical number of genetic components that interact with each other, and with a host of variable environmental factors, in the generation of the majority of major diseases. The insights of complexity that relate to connectivity, distributed control and emergent behaviour throw new light on the generation and expression of disease. They help to explain why, whatever the undoubted progress, the genomics revolution in knowledge is likely to permit us to replace our previous levels of uncertainty about the patient, only with a better defined and understood uncertainty.

Perhaps even more striking, the ideas embedded in complexity expand our understanding of a phenomenon even more mysterious than that of disease – the ever-elusive concept of health. David Aron comments that the ability of the heart to continue to function after considerable damage may be due to the redundancy of fractal structures, and that this renders them more robust and resistant to injury. He speculates that it is a loss of complexity in resting dynamics that is associated with ageing and disease.

The fashionable drive for a narrowly defined evidence-based practice is likely to accelerate trends which many of us fear: a retreat from clinical intuition to defensive documentation; from acumen to investigation; from empathic understanding to observed behaviour; from the pursuit of health to the avoidance of risk; from values-based policy to techno-managerialism.

The ideas addressed in this book, written by those who are pioneering the application of complexity theory to clinical practice, appear to provide a science-based and rigorous defence against the simplistic thinking which has impelled such dangerous trends. It is written in the spirit of the words that Bertholt Brecht put into the mouth of Galileo: that the role of the scientist is not to search for finite knowledge, but to attempt to put limits to infinite error.

This book is intended not only for clinicians who are mathematically competent, but also for the mathematically bewildered and challenged. The editor's confidence in this intention is demonstrated by his choice of one such to write this Foreword. This is an important book, it is timely and it is to be welcomed.

Marshall Marinker OBE, MD, FRCGP
Visiting Professor
Department of General Practice
Guy's, King's College and St Thomas' Hospitals
Medical and Dental School (GKT)
King's College London
May 2004

Preface

'... chance, free will and necessity — no wise incompatible — all interweavingly working together. The straight warp of necessity, not to be swerved from its ultimate course — its every alternating vibration, indeed, only tending to that; free will still free to ply her shuttle between given threads; and chance, though restrained in its play within the right lines of necessity, and sideways in its motions directed by free will, though thus prescribed to by both, chance by turns rules either, and has the last featuring blow at events.'

Herman Melville, *Moby Dick* (1851)

I begin our book with this passage from *Moby Dick*,[1] not to raise your hopes that big questions about the role of chance in human destiny will be settled by the final pages, but to remind us that these issues are by no means unique to our time. Central to the symbolism of Melville's mid-nineteenth-century classic, the complex interweaving of chance and free will against a fabric of necessity is an essentially human preoccupation, and in a world of advancing technology, increasingly important to all those who, in the broadest sense, attempt to intervene in any system to improve or modify outcomes.

Clinicians delivering healthcare at the beginning of the twenty-first century, while the target of this book, are by no means alone in the struggle to understand the dynamics of complex systems in which this combination of contingency and inevitability lead to outcomes that are often predictable only in their broadest outline, and unpredictable on a scale which makes a real difference to the lives of individuals. Evolutionary biologists still struggle with the issue of contingency in patterns of speciation and extinction; geneticists and sociologists argue over how much of our biology and behaviour arises from environmental factors, how much is genetically determined and how much a complex interweaving of both; and historians consider how much the influence of small, but in retrospect important, events such as the birth of an Alexander the Great or an Adolf Hitler have determined the political map of the world. These are all examples of complex systems with multiple, interacting components, a past and a future, evolving over time. Such systems surround us in our everyday lives as practising clinicians. What can the study of complexity offer us?

This book may not attempt to reach metaphysical conclusions, but it does address some important issues of our time. How might we understand disease mechanisms in terms of disordered dynamics? How can we adequately model the interactive nature of disease triggers? Why do patients often appear to resist well-intentioned rational advice based on sound medical research evidence? How do we harness the benefits of computerisation while safeguarding the individual needs of our patients?

This book aims to explain the foundations of the theory behind complexity, its place in clinical medicine and in the wider scientific context, using examples of its application in current and potential future medical scenarios. This is an ambitious agenda and a daunting one, were it not for the formidable team I have invited to join me in the authorship of this volume. Let me spend a few lines explaining how this book came about, and then introduce the authors.

Introductions and acknowledgements

It was purely by chance that in December 1998 I met a doctor at a meeting in London whose recent article on complexity (with social scientist David Byrne) in the *British Journal of General Practice*[2] was to kick-start the process for many of us in the United Kingdom. That doctor was Frances Griffiths, and the meeting was the launch of a new book *Clinical Futures*.[3] As a result of their paper, a group of people who had expressed an interest in it assembled at the University of Warwick the following March. Warwick is known for its association with 'chaos theory', partly because of the many writings of their mathematics professor, Ian Stewart, and his colleague Jack Cohen. Jack Cohen spoke at the meeting and a mathematician went through some fundamental theory. We all went away fairly charged with ideas and opinions, but of course few, if any, conclusions.

   The following year a smaller group of us met up at Tufton Street, Westminster, where the University of Warwick has a seminar room, and formed what became the Complexity in Primary Care Group, or 'Tufton Group' for short. Interest grew, and after several more meetings, which included speakers from different fields, we hatched the plot for an initial book. That book, *Complexity and Healthcare: an introduction*,[4] was published in 2002. By then I had developed an interest in applying these ideas to diabetes care and to health informatics, areas that will be separately explored later in this volume. The Tufton Group has an entirely informal membership, and not all of the authors of this book have any attachment to it.

Barry Tennison, author of the basic theory chapter, is an ex-research mathematician and now public health consultant to whom many of us in the group (myself included) have turned at times of need for help with the more mathematical areas of complexity. Barry is the Head of Policy and Planning at the Healthcare Commission and is an honorary professor of public health and policy at the London School of Hygiene and Tropical Medicine. I am indebted to him not only for the excellent description he has given in Chapter 2 of basic theory, but also for his support in reviewing draft manuscripts, including my own.

Paul Robinson is a general practitioner in Scarborough, North Yorkshire, a clinical senior lecturer at the University of Leeds and an education consultant to the Sowerby Centre for Health Informatics at Newcastle. Through this work he has been instrumental in the development of the PRODIGY software used as a decision support tool by clinicians all over the UK and in addition, a web-based tool for assisting general practitioners to prepare for annual appraisals. No one could be better placed to describe the role of complexity principles in decision support.

Andrew Innes is a research fellow at the University of Hull, and is studying complexity for an MD based at Warwick. As an active member of the group, one of his main areas of interest is consultation dynamics and he describes the possible insights from complexity for this area in Chapter 3.

Rachel Heath is a professor of psychology now based in New South Wales, Australia, with a strong publishing record in non-linear dynamics and has applied these principles to mental health in a powerful chapter for this book.

The final three contributors are all based in North America:

David Aron is a professor of medicine in Cleveland, Ohio, and has an interest in complexity both in clinical and organisational areas of healthcare. With both areas in mind, he will discuss the ways complexity impacts on the field of cardiology and the organisation of the coronary care unit. Cardiology is an essential field in the extension of non-linear dynamics into medicine, and his reference list contains a goldmine of sources on the theory behind this important area.

Lucila Ohno-Machado is an associate professor based at the Division of Health Sciences and Technology at Harvard Medical School and Massachusetts Institute of Technology in Boston. She is also on the faculty of the Decision Systems Group, a medical informatics laboratory based at Harvard. While trying to formulate my ideas on the use of adaptive methods for adjusting coronary heart disease risk predictions during 2002, I came across Lucila's published work and contacted her to ask for advice. She offered to co-author a paper with me, which was later published in the *British Journal of General Practice* in November 2003. In this book, we will be exploring the ways that complex pattern recognition techniques can be used to assess healthcare data.

I first got to know **Sylvie Robichaud-Ekstrand** during her visiting scholarship to the UK in 2002. Sylvie is an associate professor at the University of Montreal, and a researcher at the Montreal Heart Institute. Her work with coronary heart disease prevention provides a very practical example of how some of the core themes of this book may be applied to an increasingly important area of care.

In addition to the above, I would like to thank other colleagues interested in complexity for their advice and inspiration, particularly Frances Griffiths, Kieran Sweeney, David Kernick, Chris Burton, Hilary Hearnshaw, Tim Wilson, Trisha Greenhalgh, Paul Plsek, Sarah Fraser, Denis Pereira Gray, Krysia Saul and Iona Heath. Thank you also to Radcliffe's Gillian Nineham and Paula Moran, who have been extremely helpful in the conception and production of this book, to Alison Ray of the Scarborough Postgraduate Centre library for all her interest and help, and to my general practice partner of nine years, Ruth Pearce.

And finally, a big thank you to my family – Claire, Emma, Lauren and Brittany – for all those lost weekends.

Tim Holt
May 2004

References

1 Melville H (1851) *Moby Dick*. Oxford World's Classics (1998). Oxford University Press, Oxford.
2 Griffiths F, Byrne D (1998) General practice and the science emerging from the new theories of 'chaos' and complexity. *Br J Gen Pract*. **48**: 1697–9.
3 Marinker M, Peckham M (eds) (1998) *Clinical Futures*. BMJ Books, London.
4 Sweeney K, Griffiths F (eds) (2002) *Complexity and Healthcare: an introduction*. Radcliffe Medical Press, Oxford.

About the editor

Tim Holt is a clinical lecturer in the Centre for Primary Health Care Studies at the University of Warwick. Graduating from St George's Hospital Medical School in 1987, he first became known for co-authoring an article in the *British Medical Journal* in 1988 about the cattle disease bovine spongiform encephalopathy, a paper now widely acknowledged as an early warning of the variant CJD problem.

Since then, he has worked in both hospital medicine and primary care, most recently in rural North Yorkshire. He is a Collegiate Member of the Royal College of Physicians of London and a Fellow by Assessment of the Royal College of General Practitioners. In 2000, he was involved in the formation of the Complexity in Primary Care Group, based at Warwick, which explores the extension into healthcare of insights and concepts derived from complexity theory and non-linear dynamics. His own areas of interest within this field are diabetes care and health informatics. During his career he has particularly enjoyed collaborating with others, to promote the sharing of ideas between disciplines. He is married with three daughters, and enjoys travel, astronomy and natural history.

List of contributors

David Aron
Professor of Medicine and Epidemiology and Biostatistics
Division of Clinical and Molecular Endocrinology
Case Western Reserve University School of Medicine
Cleveland, OH, USA
and
Director
VA HSR&D Center for Quality Improvement Research
Louis Stokes Cleveland Department of Veterans Affairs Medical Center
Cleveland, OH, USA
Email: david.aron@med.va.gov

Rachel Heath
Honorary Professor
School of Behavioural Sciences
University of Newcastle
NSW, Australia
Email: rachel.heath@newcastle.edu.au

Tim A Holt
Clinical Lecturer
Centre for Primary Health Care Studies
University of Warwick
and
General Practitioner
Danby, North Yorkshire
Email: tim.holt@warwick.ac.uk

Andrew Innes
General Practitioner
Hedon, East Yorkshire
and
Research Fellow
University of Hull
Email: andrew.innes4@btopenworld.com

Lucila Ohno-Machado
Associate Professor
Division of Health Sciences and Technology
Decision Systems Group
Brigham and Women's Hospital

Harvard Medical School and
Massachusetts Institute of Technology
Boston, MA, USA
Email: machado@dsg.harvard.edu

Sylvie Robichaud-Ekstrand
Associate Professor
Faculté des Sciences Infirmières
Université de Montréal
Québec, Canada
and
Researcher
Montreal Heart Institute
Email: sylvie.robichaud-ekstrand@umontreal.ca

Paul Robinson
Honorary Senior Clinical Lecturer
Academic Unit of Primary Care
The School of Medicine
University of Leeds
and
Education Consultant
Sowerby Centre for Health Informatics
Newcastle upon Tyne
Email: paul01@btconnect.com

Barry Tennison
Head of Policy and Planning
Healthcare Commission
and
Honorary Professor of Public Health and Policy
London School of Hygiene and Tropical Medicine
Email: barry@ukph.org

PART ONE

Basic theory

CHAPTER 1

Introduction

Tim Holt

How stable and predictable are the systems we deal with in medical practice? How can this stability and predictability be quantified? How can we develop models of clinical healthcare that recognise the complex, non-linear and inter-connected nature of the real-life systems we deal with every day, and tailor our care to the individual needs of our patients?

Much of the study of complexity (and particularly the phenomenon of *chaos*) has focused on the *sensitivity* of systems to disturbing influences. This sensitivity is an example of non-linear change – a small disruption producing a much greater change in outcomes. But the reverse is also true – that in a complex, non-linear environment a large disruption may produce little, if any, effect. This will not be difficult for healthcare managers to appreciate, many of whom will have witnessed how an enormous injection of money into an area of care may not produce any discernible benefits. But how might it apply to *clinical* care?

Complex systems are made up of multiple, interconnected components and processes, interacting through non-linear relationships. When we examine biological systems, including human physiology, it is not difficult to see why such connectivity has arisen. Rather like the Internet, whose precursors were originally developed in military contexts as a network to provide resilience to the destruction of a single element, complexity is as much characterised by robustness as by vulnerability.

It is this co-existence of sensitivity and stability that characterises the systems we are dealing with in this book. Let us first take a brief look at the historical background.

I began the Preface with a passage from *Moby Dick*, published in 1851, which symbolised Melville's view of the interplay between chance, free will and pre-destination. The same decade saw the birth of a Frenchman, Henri Poincaré, who was to begin a process through which the study of non-linear dynamics could be understood in mathematical terms. Poincaré was interested in ways of modelling the movements of bodies interacting in a gravitational field (such as planets or moons), and discovered that when a *third* body is added to a system containing two gravitational bodies, the dynamics display an unusual property. The predicted trajectory of the system as a whole (i.e. the future positions of each body relative to the others) is so sensitive to measurement error in the description of the initial state, that the equations describing the system's evolution are essentially *unsolvable*. This *sensitivity to initial conditions*, even when the equations themselves are completely known and determined, is what we now call *deterministic chaos*.[1]

Imagine a catastrophe in which a violent impact occurs – say the collision of a lost space probe with a planet's surface. The final positions of each component part, scattered across the terrain, would be very difficult to predict, for obvious reasons. Their positions at impact are not known precisely, and we couldn't possibly model the interaction between the components (velocities, friction, etc.) accurately enough to produce anything more than the most rough and ready estimate of the final outcome. But this example is a single, destructive event. Now imagine that this same uncertainty exists in a situation that does not terminate, in which the same unpredictability arises for the same reason – that the initial conditions could not possibly be known in sufficient detail to predict its future state – but that continues as a healthy, robust and coherent system of connected parts, with a past and an indefinite future.

Poincaré's 'three-body problem' showed that, perhaps against intuition, this state of affairs may exist even within a system containing few components, in a system with no friction, in a system that is *closed* – one that has no exchange of energy with its external environment. If this is the case, how predictably can we expect more complex, open systems to behave as they evolve over time? Even if we could protect such systems from the effects of external disruption (an impossible task in practice), we are still faced with the unpredictability that arises *intrinsically* within the system itself, through the non-linear interactions between its components.

Ray Bradbury's 1953 book *A Sound of Thunder*[2] played on this theme and the story, if not the title, will be familiar to many. A time machine takes a group of travellers back to prehistoric times for a walk through a wood. They are told not to stray off the path, but (perhaps inevitably) one of them does, and treads on a butterfly. When the travellers return to the present, things have changed, including the result of the recent presidential election. The butterfly later became a symbol of 'chaos' for reasons that Bradbury could not have foreseen, as we shall see, and the whole issue of predictability and sensitivity to disturbance became a major focus of attention in numerous fields.

Stephen Jay Gould's 1989 book *Wonderful Life*[3] describes the fauna of the Burgess shale in Canada, a remarkable fossil bed resulting from an ancient landslide burying numerous early Cambrian creatures suddenly in low-oxygen conditions, allowing their soft parts to be preserved. Formed in exceptionally fortuitous circumstances, the shale has become something of a symbol of chance and contingency, partly because of Gould's personal interpretation of it in his book. Among the fossils we find the little animal *Pikaia*, an early example of our own phylum, the chordates. Had this phylum suffered the same fate as many of its now extinct Cambrian contemporaries, which of the subsequent developments in the history of life would still have occurred? The chordates include all the vertebrates – all the fish, frogs, dinosaurs, birds, mammals and, of course, ourselves. Would terrestrial animals, walking on four limbs and breathing air, still have arisen, perhaps in a different form? This seems very likely. Would intelligence as we know it still have evolved? Who can say?

We can't turn the clock back, rewind the tape, or in any other way repeat real-life historical experiments, to tread on a prehistoric butterfly or an ancient chordate, but using today's technology and theory we can study the dynamical properties of complex systems and measure how sensitive they are to minor disturbances. Poincaré lacked two things that only the twentieth century would bring, although both were rooted in the nineteenth century. One of these was computer technology, which has made possible the handling of the large volumes of data necessary to investigate such systems and the ability to study dynamical processes using simulations. The other was a less familiar tool: *fractal geometry*. Fractals are strange but often beautiful objects, which appear similar at different scales of magnification and are associated with the dynamical patterns of chaotic processes, in which relatively simple underlying rules generate complex structure and behaviour.

The discovery of fractals, initially as abstract mathematical confections, was followed by their appearance in all sorts of real-life scenarios. Ecologists found chaotic dynamics in the patterns of interaction between predator and prey species (most famously demonstrated in the Canadian lynx trapping figures[4]), while economists recognised similar phenomena on the stock market.[5] In both situations, their discovery marked a departure from previous models based on static equilibria to those of more dynamic states, including chaos. Meanwhile, the measles figures from the days before vaccination in North America suggested similar underlying patterns.[6] The door was opened to the application of non-linear time series analysis in a wide range of specialities. Fractal patterns were found to be the basis for many naturally occurring objects, such as coast lines, clouds, the branches of trees and, as David Aron will discuss later in this book, the structure of anatomical and physiological systems, including cardiac conduction tissue and the patterns of electrical activity within it. This has led to the conclusion that chaotic processes are, perhaps counter-intuitively, a healthy sign of normality in these systems. One reason for this might be that such structures are physiologically efficient and therefore adaptive in the sense of high selection value, but also that they enable complex structures to arise through the application and iteration of very simple rules in the development of living forms. This may go some way to explain the otherwise baffling complexity that arises during the embryological development of a multicellular organism.

Perhaps the most famous application of this new 'chaos theory' as it became called (although we should be clear that chaos is a *phenomenon*, not a theory in itself), occurred in the study of weather patterns. In 1963, the meteorologist Edward Lorenz published a landmark paper[7] in which he described an abstract model of a simplified weather system involving just three variables, three model parameters and three equations. Echoing Poincaré's three-body problem, the model demonstrated that even when the system is *entirely deterministic* (the equations specify precise outputs for given inputs) and 'simple' in the sense that only three variables were involved, the system's behaviour cannot be predicted beyond a few steps into the future, because of the amplification of tiny uncertainties in the initial conditions. While real-life weather systems are much more complex than this, the demonstration of low-dimensional chaos in Lorenz's model set a limit on the future success of weather forecasting. In the time since this paper was published, forecasting has become much more successful in the very short term (through improvements in the technology of barometry, etc.), but the distance into the future that reliable predictions can be made has changed very little. Weather forecasters are only too aware of this. However obsessively they measure the initial starting conditions, their 'predictive time horizon' into the future is inevitably short. It is limited by the *geometry* of weather dynamics, and not by inadequate measurement techniques.

Lorenz recognised that when one of his variables is plotted as a time series, no discernible pattern is present and the variation is effectively random (Figure 1.1).

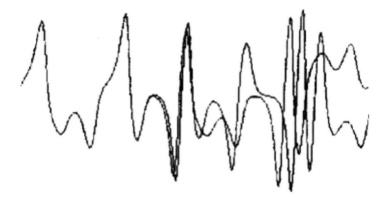

Figure 1.1 A time series of just one of Lorenz's variables. The diagram demonstrates a lack of apparent pattern, difficult to distinguish from random variation. It also demonstrates 'sensitivity to initial conditions', in that a tiny uncertainty introduced early on in the profile has led to diverging trajectories that begin running in similar directions but after a while bear no correlation to each other. (www.bath.ac.uk/~ma1jnr/html%20webpage/edward_lorenz.html)

It would be difficult to guess that such a pattern is generated by a relatively simple deterministic system.

But when the other two variables are included as a *phase space* diagram (*see* Figure 1.2), the underlying order is revealed. This was a crucial insight uncovered by Lorenz's work, and his weather system's butterfly-shaped attractor has become an enduring symbol of chaos. For a dynamic representation in real time visit www.sat.t.u-tokyo.ac.jp/~hideyuki/java/Attract.html

A *phase space* diagram plots the values of each variable as separate axes. The current state of the system is represented by a point in this space, and as time passes, the point becomes a 'trajectory' as the value of each variable changes. The system may be restricted to a certain region and pattern in phase space – the system's attractor. The dynamics of the system can be studied by examining the geometrical properties of the attractor. In a chaotic system, the structure is typically fractal, with self-similar structure at all scales, and while the overall pattern is stable, nearby trajectories tend to diverge from close starting points (representing similar initial conditions), limiting predictability to a short time horizon.

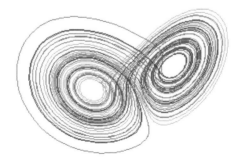

Figure 1.2 Plotted in 'phase space', the Lorenz data reveal the system's more orderly underlying attractor (http://psychology.unn.ac.uk/dick/Chaos/Dynamics.htm). The attractor has fractal properties: a slice through one of its 'wings' could be magnified to reveal self-similar structure at different scales.

What use are these insights to clinicians?

First of all, we might identify scenarios in which underlying order goes unrecognised because of the apparent randomness on the surface, particularly when one variable is assessed in isolation. In Chapter 5, I will explore the possibility that type 1 diabetes is such a scenario and discuss how this might help in assisting patients to achieve tight glycaemic control. Second, we may recognise fractal patterns in physiological systems and thereby access new ways of measuring the health of the system according to such properties. This approach, using non-linear time series analysis, may also help us identify disorders that are essentially dynamical in origin. Finally, we may recognise that even when the number of variables in a system is reduced to just a few, non-linearity may limit predictability and our ability to control outcomes. The *interactions* between component variables, when non-linear, cannot be handled as easily as the variables themselves by simply taking 'averages', and standard analytical approaches (which work well in situations where components are independent and linearly related to outcomes) become unworkable.[8]

But clearly, not all outcomes in complex systems are unpredictable and not all trajectories diverge. Indeed, some surprising examples of 'convergence' are readily seen in all sorts of scenarios. Evolution has frequently produced 'analogous' forms and functions in unrelated species, such as the very similar body plans of marsupial and placental mammals. Identical twins reared in different childhood environments may develop remarkably similar personality traits as adults.[9] And outcomes in political history may display a similar broad-brush convergence while contingency dictates the details, so that agriculture, animal domestication, writing, and human settlement have all arisen independently in numerous centres worldwide at different times.[10]

The next chapter provides a more technical description of the theory behind complexity and provides references through which further information can be accessed. Some readers may find this section difficult and may wish to take each chapter at a time, relying on the theoretical explanations that each author has given independently for his or her own area. But one issue central to the book that is worth discussing before proceeding further is the use of the term 'complexity' itself. What do we mean by complexity? How do complex systems differ from those that are merely complicated? And what is meant by the term '*complex adaptive system*'?

Definitions of complexity

We all have an intuitive understanding of what it means for a system to be complex. But can we define the term any more precisely? This problem may be tackled from a number of different angles, typically taking into account:

- the number of component variables in the system (the systems *dimension*)
- the degree of *connectivity* between the components
- the dynamical properties and *regularity* of the system's behaviour
- the information content and *compressibility* of data generated by the system.

Later in this book Rachel Heath discusses various ways of measuring complexity in time series data, including the correlation dimension D_2, and the approximate entropy ApEn. Approximate entropy is a measure of irregularity in a time series dataset and is low in relatively simple regular systems, rising with increasing complexity as the order in the system becomes less apparent.

The dynamical repertoire of non-linear systems includes a spectrum of behaviours from the *point attractor*, where all the variables tend to return to baseline values at an equilibrium position in phase space; through more dynamic but still orderly patterns such as *periodicity*, where a sequence of values of the variables is repeated recurrently; to *chaos*, where the system keeps moving through a series of values that neither settle down to a steady state nor repeat themselves. Chaotic behaviour may be predictable indefinitely in its broad outline because the values of the variables are bounded and the system contains an attractor (the Lorenz attractor discussed above is an example). It is predictable in the very short term because the trajectories of similar starting conditions initially move through phase space in similar directions before departing. But in the medium term it is impossible to say exactly where the system will be found in terms of the values of the component variables. As Rachel Heath notes, any of these behaviours may be contaminated by *random noise*. Pure noise is essentially without structure in phase space and is therefore completely unpredictable, as there is no tendency for trajectories to move in similar directions locally.

The *dimension* of noise is infinite, and here is a possible dilemma. If we are to assume that a rise in the dimensions of a system indicates a rise in complexity (an apparently safe assumption as we introduce more component variables to a simple system, as Poincaré proposed with the gravitational bodies), we see the behaviour getting increasingly close to the dynamics of random noise by this criterion. So is random noise simply an ultimate state of complexity that represents a dimensionality too high to be measured? Or are our attempts to define complexity purely in terms of the system's dimension flawed?

Gary Flake finds a satisfying solution to this problem, by using the term '*effective complexity*'.[11] Taking a computer science perspective, Flake clarifies the issue by measuring complexity using both the information content and the *compressibility* of the data associated with the system of interest. A dataset is compressible if an algorithm exists that can reproduce or generate the data, an algorithm that is simpler than the data itself. Imagine a dataset containing a long string of zeros:

$$000000000000000000000000000000000000000$$

Such a string contains virtually no information. Now imagine a string of values that oscillate periodically between 0 and 1:

$$010101010101010101010101010101010101010$$

This string contains more, but still little information. Next consider the first 15 numbers in the Fibonacci sequence, generated by adding the last two values together to produce the next number:

$$1, 1, 2, 3, 5, 8, 13, 21, 34, 55, 89, 144, 233, 377, 610$$

Such a series is produced by a very simple algorithm. The pattern is still relatively orderly, contains little information and is evident in the first few numbers. As a means of coding an encrypted message, this algorithm would not be very useful, although more so than the two sequences before it. At the other end of the spectrum there is (by definition) no algorithm that can generate a series of truly random numbers. A computer may contain in its memory a list of random numbers and it may be easy to calculate their parameters (such as the mean and the standard deviation), but a random dataset is not computable in the usual sense as no algorithm could generate the data in finite time.

What about chaotic data, which superficially resemble random data? A chaotic time series can be generated using an algorithm – we have seen this discussed above using the example of the Lorenz attractor, a highly complex object generated by a remarkably simple set of equations. And yet this data appears random. Let's take a series of data from the Lorenz paper,[7] which represents the values of one of the system's variables over time:

0075, 0076, 0082, 0069, −0079, −0077, −0083, −0073,

−0074, 0079, 0072, −0077, 0072

This series may appear to vary randomly, but as we have seen, there is an underlying pattern evident not only in the visible structure of the attractor, but also in the existence of just three equations that determine the system's behaviour. This pattern reflects the underlying order in the system but is difficult, if not impossible, to discern when only one variable is measured in isolation.

At which end of the compressibility spectrum do the Lorenz data lie? The answer is that they lie somewhere in the middle, because while the dataset can be

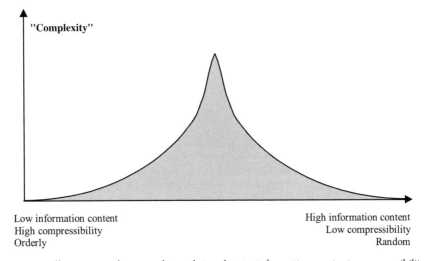

"Complexity"

Low information content	High information content
High compressibility	Low compressibility
Orderly	Random

Figure 1.3 Effective complexity and its relationship to information content, compressibility and order (after Flake). Flake makes a good case that most of the interesting things that happen in nature exist in the middle ground between computability and incomputability, but his argument is beyond the scope of this book. © MIT Press. Adapted with permission from Flake GW (2000) *The Computational Beauty of Nature: computer explorations of fractals, chaos, complex systems, and adaptation.* MIT Press, Cambridge, MA.

produced by a simple computer algorithm, its infinitely detailed fractal structure cannot be computed in finite time. It is therefore only *partially computable* and lies in the middle ground between low and high compressibility, the area that Flake identifies with maximum effective complexity (Figure 1.3).

The recognition of this 'middle ground' that lies between highly ordered and random states has become an important insight in the application of complexity theory to all sorts of areas. It is this same area that Kauffman identifies with the 'edge of chaos',[12] an area where, dynamically and morphologically, living systems exist and harness *self-organisation* as a source of order. It is the area that Stacey identifies as the 'complex zone' lying between the extremes of high and low agreement and certainty in management scenarios (see Chapter 3). It is the region in which economies thrive between 'frozen' equilibrium states of decreasing investment returns and the more disorderly and unstable behaviour associated with positive feedback, increasing returns and speculative bubbles.[5]

Complexity and connectivity

Clearly, the *connections* between the components of a system are an important determinant of the system's complexity. How might this connectivity be quantified and studied?

Stuart Kauffman uses as one of his fundamental tools a model he calls *NK landscapes*.[12] If there are N components in a system and each is influenced by K other components, then we can investigate the properties of the system by 'tuning' the K parameter. This model might apply to a genotype in which there are N genes determining the organism's fitness, with the fitness contribution of each gene influenced by K other genes. A 'fitness landscape' can then be constructed in which the overall fitness is plotted as an axis within the space of possible gene combinations.

In the many studies Kauffman has applied to this model, we again see that there is an *optimum range of values* of K that produce the most interesting behaviour. When K has a very low value relative to N nothing very interesting happens and the fitness landscape is smooth, indicating a close correlation between the fitness values of similar gene combinations, i.e. combinations lying close to each other in the landscape. At the other extreme, where K has its maximum value of $N - 1$, the structure of the landscape is effectively random, or *uncorrelated* – two points close by in the landscape are no more likely to be of similar fitness than two more distant points. Between these extremes, the landscapes display complex structure that is 'rugged' but correlated. It is on such landscapes that evolution occurs in real biological systems, where the K parameter may represent the interactions between genes, or the relationships between co-evolving species in an ecosystem. Fitness landscapes and their possible extension to risk factor management in medicine will be discussed again in Chapter 10.

So whichever index we choose – dimensionality, compressibility, information content or connectivity – we see that the most interesting, creative and complex behaviour requires a compromise between extremes, a middle ground. This allows an important conceptual distinction to be made between systems that are *complex* and those that are merely *complicated*.

Complex adaptive systems

Complex adaptive systems (CAS) are characterised by the following key properties (see also Holland[8]):

1 They consist of multiple component 'agents' that are connected through local agent–agent interactions.
2 These interactions tend to be *non-linear* and *feedback* on one another.
3 Boundaries, both between the system and its environment, and between the internal compartments, are indistinct and *dynamic.*
4 Energy and other resources are extracted from the environment and are continuously dissipated, keeping the system *'far from equilibrium'.* There is a turnover of components, but structure and information are preserved over time.
5 The system can *adapt* to changes in the internal and external environment.
6 There is *overlap* between subcategories of agent in the system, so that an individual agent may belong to more than one subcategory.
7 Because of this connectivity, fuzzy boundaries and overlap it is difficult to simply remove a part of the system and replace it.
8 The system has a *history,* which determines its current structure, internal organisation and behaviour, so that it is capable of *learning.*
9 Emergent properties may arise through the lower-level interactions between agents. Such properties cannot be understood at the level of the agents themselves.

These properties might apply to a range of system types, including a living organism, an immune system within it, a human organisation, an economy, or an ecosystem. Andrew Innes discusses CAS in the context of the consultation on page 45, and David Aron in terms of coronary care organisation on page 61. As an example, let us look at the human brain, the most complex system known.

The brain consists of about 100 billion individual 'agents' – in this case neurones – that interact with each other through synaptic connections. Chemical signals pass a very short distance across these connections from one neurone to the next. (The neurones also interact through hormonal and other mediators that are less localised.) Neurones vary over time in their responsiveness to stimulation. The mechanisms through which the brain 'learns' are still poorly understood and beyond the scope of this book. However, in the 1940s, Hebb proposed that a very simple rule underlying synaptic firing would allow past patterns of stimulation to alter the receptiveness of neurones to future stimulation.[13] Quite simply, he suggested that if a synapse had been successful in the past at making a neurone fire, the receptivity of that neurone to subsequent stimulation by that synapse would be increased. The individual neurones themselves have no cognitive capacity, but relatively simple non-linear interactions between them may generate higher-level cognitive functions.

Another important feature of the brain that is frequently seen in complex systems is a dependence on *distributed* pattern recognition. The brain is massively parallel, recognising patterns by responding to multiple stimuli distributed across different areas of cortex. While localised areas have specific functions, some of which are more essential to cognition than others, no single area is 'in command'. There is, of course, a higher structure to the functional domains of the brain, but the sensation of a continuous stream of consciousness occurring in some well localised 'central processing unit' appears to be an illusion: *the brain has no CPU*. This area is discussed further in Chapter 7 by Paul Robinson in the context of decision making.

In his book *Emergence*,[14] Steven Johnson describes a similar form of decentralisation in ant colonies, and names one of his chapters 'The Myth of the Ant Queen'. A colony does indeed have a queen ant, but the behaviour of the colony and its 'intelligence' are distributed phenomena evolving over timescales that exceed the lifetime of individual ants, and are not a result of the queen's 'control'. The emergent properties of the colony (such as the ability to maintain a stable internal temperature within the nest) arise through the interactions between the ants via pheromone signals. The information 'learned' by the system as a whole is in this case stored in the patterns of these signals rather than in neuronal connections, but the mechanisms are otherwise similar in that they depend on historical patterns of information stored in the interrelationships between agents.

So how does all this apply to clinical medicine?

In Chapter 5, I explore the implications of non-linear dynamics for patients with diabetes, trying to predict the behaviour of their own individual trajectory through a space of possible values for the determinants of blood glucose. Rachel Heath discusses how a number of psychiatric illnesses may be understood in terms of disordered dynamics, arising intrinsically from within the system (Chapter 6). And David Aron gives an account of the insights gained through an understanding of complex non-linear mechanisms in the functioning of the cardiovascular system in both health and disease (Chapter 4). He shows that the same principles might apply at all levels of the system, from the individual cell to the healthcare organisation. In other chapters, we explore the implications for patient care and decision support in a consultation environment where research evidence is increasingly available to both patient and clinician, but the use of this evidence and its conversion into clinical benefits is a complex process that must recognise the multidimensional, and not always rational, agendas of all the parties concerned. We also look at how electronic healthcare databases, themselves dynamic, evolving repositories of information, can be assessed to recognise and adapt to changing patterns of clinical need during the coming decades, offering patients the benefits both of the current 'best evidence' and the lessons learnt through the healthcare system's past experiences. And we give examples of how these principles can be put into practice in the delivery of clinical healthcare.

References

1   Stewart I (1997) *Does God Play Dice?* (2e). Penguin, London.
2   Bradbury R (1953) A Sound of Thunder. In: *Stories of Ray Bradbury*, Vol. 1, (1983). Granada, St Albans.
3   Gould SJ (1989) *Wonderful Life: the Burgess shale and the nature of history.* Penguin, London.

4   Schaffer WM (1986) Order and chaos in ecological systems. *Ecology.* **66**(1): 93–106.

5   Waldrop MM (1992) *Complexity.* Simon and Schuster, New York.

6   Schaffer WM (1985) Can non-linear dynamics elucidate mechanisms in ecology and epidemiology? *IMA Journal of Mathematics Applied in Medicine and Biology.* **2**: 221–52.

7   Lorenz E (1963) Deterministic non-periodic flow. *Journal of the Atmospheric Sciences.* **20**: 130–41.

8   Holland JH (1996) *Hidden Order: how adaptation builds complexity.* Perseus Books, Cambridge, MA, pp. 15–23.

9   Pinker S (1998) *How the Mind Works.* Allen Lane (Penguin), London, pp. 20–1.

10 Diamond J (1998) *Guns, Germs and Steel.* Random House (Vintage), London.

11 Flake GW (1998) *The Computational Beauty of Nature: computer explorations of fractals, chaos, complex systems, and adaptation.* MIT Press, Cambridge, MA.

12 Kauffman SA (1993) *The Origins of Order: self-organisation and selection in evolution.* Oxford University Press, New York.

13 Hebb DO (1949) *The Organisation of Behaviour: a neuropsychological theory.* Wiley, New York, p. 62.

14 Johnson S (2002) *Emergence.* Penguin, London.

CHAPTER 2

Basic theory

Barry Tennison

Introduction

This chapter aims to explain, in fairly technical terms, the basic theory behind complexity, providing the more mathematically minded reader with a basic understanding, and with references that can be consulted for further details.

It begins with one of the most fundamental principles that underpins complexity, both conceptually and in the practical sense required to model complex systems and understand their dynamics: the meanings of *linearity* and *non-linearity*. I then discuss insights from dynamical systems theory and statistical mechanics, and their relevance to complexity, using simple examples. This will take us on to *fractal geometry*, and it relationship to the dynamics of *chaotic* behaviour.

Linearity and non-linearity

The terms 'linear' and 'non-linear' are often used by those interested in complexity. The words are usually being applied, implicitly or explicitly, to a description or model of a system. The usages seem to fall into two main groups:

- mathematical usage
- less mathematical or informal usage.

There is some danger of misunderstanding or confusion when these two are not distinguished. They are described below, and some connections and distinctions made.

The mathematical usage of 'linear' and 'non-linear'

The mathematical usage is quite precise, and concerns functions, maps or relationships between variables. The simplest example is in a relationship between two variables x and y. If there is a constant number a such that

$$y = ax \tag{1}$$

(where the expression on the right means a times x), then the relationship between x and y is (strictly) linear. This means that, for example, if x increases by 20%, then

y increases by 20%: a proportionate change in x causes the same proportionate change in y.

Many scientists (but not pure mathematicians) would say that the relationship between x and y is linear if there are constants a and b such that:

$$y = ax + b. \tag{2}$$

This is because the relationship is still 'of degree 1' in x, as opposed to say:

$$y = ax^2 + b \tag{3}$$

where the involvement of x (as x squared) is of degree 2 in x (this is an example of a non-linear relationship; see below). However, note that in (2), a proportionate increase in x does not, if $b \neq 0$, lead to a proportionate increase in y (try it by taking for example $a = 3$, $b = 70$, $x = 10$, and then increase x by 20%). Some pure mathematicians (especially geometers) would call a relationship of type (2) *affine* rather than linear.[1]

As we shall see below, systems often involve many more than two variables, and mathematically this corresponds to using higher-dimensional spaces in our models. A typical linear relationship would then be:

$$y = \sum_{i=1}^{n} a_i x_i \tag{4}$$

where the x_i are the 'independent variables' and y is the 'dependent variable'. Here n is the dimension of the space of the x_i, and the a_i are constants. More generally, there may also be many ys, and this then looks like:

$$y_j = \sum_{i=1}^{n} a_{ji} x_i \tag{5}$$

or more succinctly:

$$y = Ax \tag{6}$$

where now both y and x are vectors and A is a matrix (or a linear operator, depending on how you look at it).

Once things get this complicated, mathematicians characterise linear relationships differently. They start to talk about vector spaces (say X and Y) and a map between them:

$$X \xrightarrow{f} Y \quad \text{[we write } y = f(x) \text{ for } x \text{ in } X \text{ and } y \text{ in } Y]. \tag{7}$$

This f is then said to be linear if it satisfies the generalisation of the 'increase by 20%' property mentioned above. For completeness, and because as we shall see below they are vital, the conditions[2] are:

$$\text{for all } x \text{ and } x' \text{ in } X, \quad f(x + x') = f(x) + f(x') \tag{8}$$

and

$$\text{for all } x \text{ in } X \text{ and real numbers } \lambda, \quad f(\lambda x) = \lambda f(x). \tag{9}$$

The second condition is essentially the 'proportionality' property mentioned above. More generally, the λ in (9) might range through all complex numbers, or more generally any field (a special kind of mathematical object) over which the vector spaces X and Y are defined. Increasing levels of generality allow the linear spaces to be infinite dimensional. The first condition (8) is a 'superposition' condition, of which we shall see more below.

This leads to probably the most general version of pure mathematical 'linearity'. A map f from X to Y is linear if both X and Y have a linear structure (this can be defined precisely) and the map f satisfies the equivalent of conditions (8) and (9) above. The spaces X and Y might be vector spaces of finite or infinite dimension (they would be of infinite dimension in many applications in quantum theory).

People sometimes talk instead of a linear *system*, which is conceived of as a 'black box' with an input and an output (Figure 2.1). To say this is linear is to say that the output changes in proportion to the input, and (more subtly and sometimes more difficult to formalise) that superposition applies: if input x gives output y, and input x' gives output y', then input $x + x'$ gives output $y + y'$. These conditions correspond to (9) and (8) respectively.

What then, in mathematics, is non-linearity? At a first acquaintance, one would guess that it was any relationship that did not satisfy the linearity conditions. However, for well-established reasons, mathematicians prefer to use the negative term more inclusively: a non-linear relationship or system is one that *does not necessarily* satisfy the linearity conditions (but may do so). This prevents one from having to make artificial distinctions. In this sense, the non-linear includes the linear.

Simple examples of non-linear connections between variables might include:

$$y = ax^2 + bx + c \quad \text{[note that this } is \text{ linear if } a = c = 0\text{]} \tag{10}$$

$$y = \sqrt{x} \tag{11}$$

$$y = \exp(x) \tag{12}$$

$$y = kx(1 - x) \quad \text{[this is one form of the logistic equation}^3\text{]} \tag{13}$$

as well as those defined implicitly by a connection between x and y rather than by an equation giving y directly in terms of x; for example:

$$y^3 + x^3 = xy \tag{14}$$

$$\frac{dy}{dx} = y \tag{15}$$

$$\dot{x} = ax - cxy \quad \text{and} \quad \dot{y} = -by + dxy \tag{16}$$

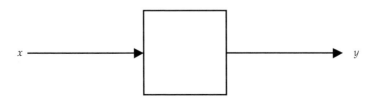

Figure 2.1 System as a black box.

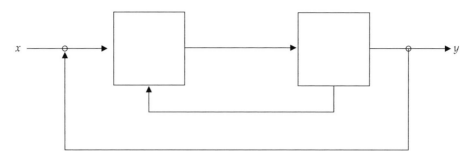

Figure 2.2 Non-linearity arising from feedback.

For good reasons, although possibly initially confusingly, (15) is called a linear differential equation, whereas (16) is a first-order non-linear system of equations (x with a dot over it denotes differentiation with respect to the unmentioned variable t: with t interpreted as time, this is the simplest predator–prey model). It is non-linear because of the occurrence of the term xy where x and y are multiplied together.

More involved are algorithmic relationships, which cannot be expressed in terms of a single equation. One example would be the yes/no decision to shock (output) by an automated defibrillator, where the inputs are the various measurements it takes. Another example would be the computations that turn a number representing a plaintext into a ciphertext in cryptography.[4]

Similarly, a non-linear system is any black box like Figure 2.1, where we do not assume the proportionality and superposition conditions. One way in which non-linear systems arise naturally is by being made up of subsystems with feedback loops, as in Figure 2.2. Even if the subsystems are each linear, the total system need not be (although it can be in some cases).

After seeing this brief handful of non-linear maps and systems, why would one want to restrict oneself to considering only linear maps or systems? The answer is, first that linear maps and systems are much easier to handle; and second, that any (non-linear) map or system can be *approximated* by linear systems. To elaborate the first point, there are many techniques available to analyse linear maps and systems, for example matrix algebra, decomposition theorems and theories, spectral analysis and explicit solutions in terms of known maps or functions. These often give a practically complete description of the system (which may still be very complicated).

The second point has been a fundamental achievement and success of applying mathematics in many branches of science. In its geometric essence, this is always about having a problem described by a point on a geometric object (like a curve, surface or higher-dimensional manifold) and saying that near that point the object can be treated as if it was linear (or flat) – think of the tangent line to a curve, or the tangent plane to a surface. For example:

- differential calculus is a spectacularly successful way of approximating a function by a linear function, and then approximating the error in doing this by another linear function, and so on
- many highly successful statistical methods, like multilinear regression and generalised linear models, arise essentially from applying a linear approximation to an arbitrary (non-linear) model – think of regression lines showing significant

or non-significant associations between variables with random components: the computation of the regression line assumes a linear model around the mean of the data points
- perturbation theory in quantum mechanics[5] applies linear approximations to non-linear situations; the fact that it does or does not 'work' (for example, converge) in any particular problem reveals much about the extent to which the approximation is valid.

The linear problem is then usually much more tractable, and describes the system *locally* near the point. Further insight is gained by distinguishing the *local* properties of the problem from the *global* properties – those which arise further away from the point in question.

In considering complex systems, the most immediately relevant mathematical models are those of dynamical systems theory.[6,7] Some of the concepts and results that come from dynamical systems theory are:

- phase space
- trajectories or orbits
- attractors
- structural stability
- local versus global properties ('all dynamical systems are locally linear').

See the next section (pp. 21–8) for some explanation and examples of dynamical systems theory and its applications in complexity theory.

The less mathematical or informal usage of 'linear' and 'non-linear'

The non-mathematical use of the words 'linear' and 'non-linear' are rather harder to pin down with any precision. The Shorter Oxford English Dictionary (1993 edition) gives six definitions for 'linear', most of which are about resemblance to a (straight?) line. In addition to the mathematical one, there is also:

- progressing in a single direction by regular steps or stages, sequential.

The corresponding definition of non-linear reads:

- not linear; not pertaining to, involving or arranged in a (straight) line
- involving a lack of linearity between two related quantities such as input and output.

In the world of complexity theory, these meanings are both extended and made less precise. For example, to quote an online glossary:

- linear systems are ones where the result of a change is, by and large, predictable
- non-linear systems are ones where the results of changing one factor are unpredictable but are still replicable. Sometimes a small change in *a* results in no change in *b*, other times a huge change in *b*.[8]

Cilliers[9] offers some insight into the non-mathematical use of non-linearity:

- [A precondition for self-organisation is that] the interactions among units have to be *non-linear*. Small changes must be able to cause large effects, and the combination of patterns should result in the formation of new ones, not merely in linear combinations of the constituents.[10]
- ... the magnifying power of non-linearity.[11]
- Any proper language consists of a large number of words whose meanings are constituted through their relationships with each other ... In these relationships non-linearity and asymmetry are of vital importance.[12]
- A large system of linear elements can usually be collapsed into an equivalent system that is very much smaller. Non-linearity ... guarantees that small causes can have large results and vice versa. It is a precondition for complexity.[13]

This idea that in a non-linear system, small inputs can lead to large outputs while large inputs can lead to small outputs, seems to be at the core of many non-mathematical concepts of non-linearity. It is important to note that in a linear system, small inputs can have large results (think of $y = 1000000 * x$), but large inputs having small effects *in the same system* is evidence of non-linearity.

One danger of confining one's sense of linearity to this '*proportionality*' (compare (9) above) is that one misses the essential second component, that of *superposition* (see (8) above and the nearby discussion of linear systems). Holland expresses a version of this:

> Emergence is above all a product of coupled, context-dependent interactions. Technically, these interactions, and the resulting system are *non-linear*: the behaviour of the overall system *cannot* be obtained by *summing* the behaviours of the individual parts.[14]

For Nicholis, it is the core of non-linearity:

> A striking difference between linear and nonlinear laws is whether the property of superposition holds or breaks down. In a linear system the ultimate effect of the combined action of two different causes is merely the superposition of the effects of each cause taken individually. But in a nonlinear system adding two elementary actions to one another can induce dramatic new effects reflecting the onset of cooperativity between the constituent elements. This can give rise to unexpected structures and events whose properties can be quite different from those of the underlying elementary laws, in the form of abrupt transitions, a multiplicity of states, pattern formation, or an irregular markedly unpredictable evolution in space and time referred to as deterministic chaos. Nonlinear science is, therefore, the science of evolution and complexity.[15]

Finally, there are some mathematical concepts which are related to but essentially different from linearity and non-linearity:

- continuous versus discontinuous[16] (think of a piece of elastic breaking)
- structurally stable versus structurally unstable[17] (does a small perturbation of the parameters or definition of the system lead to small or to dramatic changes in its overall dynamics — see the example of the ideal and non-ideal pendulum below).

In some informal uses of the words 'linear' and 'non-linear' there seems to be potential for confusion with these very different concepts.

Conclusion on linearity and non-linearity

We have seen that the terms 'linear' and 'non-linear' are used differently by different people and in different fields of study and intellectual traditions. Although this richness can be valuable, it is important to be sure of the sense in which the words are being used. In particular, one must be careful in applying the results of one field to another where not only the meanings and definitions may differ, but also the preconditions for the conclusions may be misunderstood. Very informal uses ('that's non-linear thinking!') should be treated as such.

Dynamical systems: theory and examples

In considering complex systems, the most immediately relevant mathematical models are those of dynamical systems theory.[6,18] The aim of this section is to give an accessible introduction to this theory, mainly through examples. Some of the concepts and results of dynamical systems theory are very relevant to complexity:

- phase space
- trajectories or orbits
- attractors
- structural stability
- local versus global properties ('all dynamical systems are locally linear').

Dynamical systems theory is quite a complicated theory, and fairly unapproachable for those without a substantial mathematical training. It includes precise definitions and elaborations of very fundamental concepts such as phase space, attractors and structural stability. It is hard to gain a good understanding of the strangeness and power of complexity theory without having some grasp of these concepts.

Rather than describe dynamical systems theory mathematically, I have chosen to present some simple examples that illustrate some of the main points. It is important to note that even quite simple examples can show some interesting features which illustrate what may happen in more complicated, real-world systems.

The first, quite simple, example starts out with an idealised pendulum (Figure 2.3). This has a light, thin, rigid rod, fixed at one end to a pivot, with a frictionless joint allowing motion in only one plane (note that the rod is rigid, not a piece of string: the reason should soon become apparent). At the other end, there is a heavy weight (the bob). The bob is so heavy that we idealise the rod to have zero

Figure 2.3 The simple pendulum.

weight, and we assume to start with that the pendulum is in a vacuum, so that there is no air resistance, nor any forces other than gravity acting on it.

The state this pendulum is in at any particular time t is completely determined by two values: one describing the position of the bob, and the other describing its velocity. We call these two variables x and y, as in the diagram. The physics of the situation can be used to tell us that the following equation holds:

$$\frac{dy}{dt} = -c\sin(x) \tag{17}$$

where sin is the trigonometric sine function, and c is a constant which depends on the length of the rod and the strength of gravity. Additionally, since y is the rate of change of lx (where l is the length of the rod), we have:

$$l\frac{dx}{dt} = y \tag{18}$$

and these two equations completely define the behaviour of the system.

The pendulum is a simple dynamical system. The equations describe and define how the motion of the pendulum evolves with time. If we start the pendulum at time t with specific values of x and y, the equation shows what values of x and y then follow as t increases (that is, as time passes). For example, if we start with the rod horizontally extended to the right ($x = 90°$, $y = 0$) and the bob not moving (by using a hand to lift the bob to the required position), then the equation shows (unsurprisingly) that the pendulum will swing clockwise until the rod is horizontal to the left ($x = -90°$, $y = 0$) and then swing back to the original position, and it will go on doing this forever. This perpetual motion is due to the idealised assumptions of no friction and no air resistance; those offended by this should wait until later when we see what happens when we remove these assumptions.

The dynamical systems theory approach to a system like this is to consider its *phase space*. This is an abstract space in which all the *states* of the system can be plotted. For the pendulum, this is the two-dimensional space with coordinates x and y: the state of the pendulum is completely described by these two values. On this two-dimensional coordinate plane we can plot paths (or *trajectories*, also known as *orbits*) which show how the state of the system evolves with time. The resulting diagram is shown in Figure 2.4.

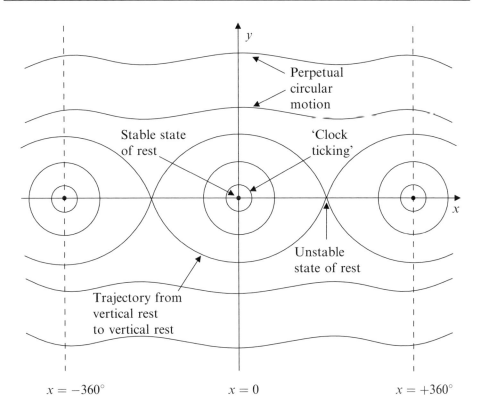

Figure 2.4 Phase space for idealised pendulum.

Some readers may be familiar with an elementary mathematical treatment of the pendulum, which limits attention to when the swings are small. Then x is small, so $\sin(x)$ can be approximated by x, giving the linear equations:

$$\frac{dy}{dt} = -cx \tag{19}$$

$$l\frac{dx}{dt} = y \tag{20}$$

which can be solved exactly. This pays attention only to the centre of the phase space, where the trajectories are approximately circular. This is in fact the *linear approximation* (see earlier section on linearity and non-linearity) to the system around the point $x = 0°$, $y = 0$, where the pendulum hangs vertically downwards and motionless.

Let us make a simple visual change to illuminate the case of the idealised pendulum. First, note that the values of x actually repeat every 360° (for example, 90° describes the same physical position as does $450° = 90° + 360°$). Accordingly, the pattern of trajectories repeats every 360° in the x direction. So we can cut the sheet along the vertical lines $x = -180°$ and $x = 180°$, throw away the duplicates and glue the two vertical lines together, to get a diagram of trajectories on a cylinder (Figure 2.5).

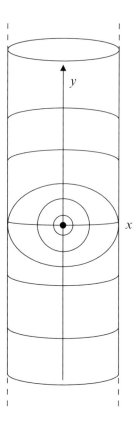

Figure 2.5 Idealised pendulum: phase space as a cylinder.

If we now take this cylinder and bend it into a u-tube (Figure 2.6), almost miraculously, the trajectories now look more regular — they are just the horizontal sections (or 'cuts') through the u-tube. Indeed, the vertical direction now represents the total energy (kinetic plus potential) of the system, and the trajectories are curves where the energy remains constant, due to our idealised assumptions of no friction or air resistance.

On the u-tube, the trajectories fall into five types:

(a) the circles around one arm of the u-tube: these correspond to the pendulum spinning round and round the pivot

(b) the 'figure-of-eight' across the top of the u-tube: this corresponds to the pendulum swinging up to the vertical position and just remaining poised there

(c) the more or less circular curves around the bend of the u-tube: these correspond to the pendulum making periodic swings to and fro (to different heights for different trajectories)

(d) the point at the top of the u-tube: this is the unstable equilibrium with the pendulum vertical

(e) the point at the bottom of the u-tube: this is the stable equilibrium with the pendulum motionless and hanging vertically down.

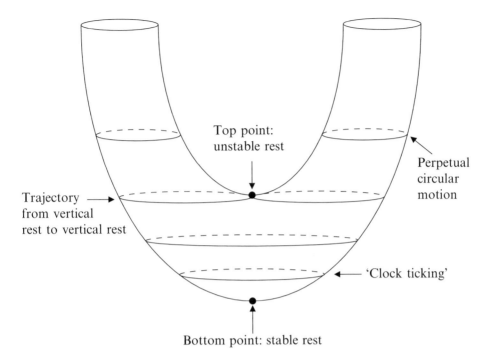

Figure 2.6 Idealised pendulum: phase space as a u-tube.

One great advantage of the u-tube representation is that we can now see what happens when we remove our ideal assumptions. If the pivot has friction or air resists the motion, this is equivalent to there being an energy drain on the system. Visualise this as a little tap at the lowest point of the u-tube, leaking energy. This changes the pattern of trajectories to look like Figure 2.7.

The trajectories now fall into four very different types:

(a′) those which twirl around one of the arms of the u-tube, and descend to end up at the bottom point: these correspond to the pendulum spinning round and round the pivot, slowing to swing to and fro, with the swing getting smaller and smaller until the pendulum comes to rest hanging down

(b′) those which twirl around one of the arms of the u-tube, and descend to end up at the top point of the u-tube: these correspond to the pendulum spinning round and round the pivot, slowing until the pendulum comes to rest at the unstable equilibrium with the pendulum vertical

(c′) the point at the top of the u-tube: this is the unstable equilibrium with the pendulum vertical

(d′) the point at the bottom of the u-tube: this is the stable equilibrium with the pendulum motionless and hanging vertically down.

This is a very dramatic change in the pattern of trajectories. As we shall see below, this shows that the idealised pendulum is not a structurally stable system.

The pendulum example can be varied to give more complex behaviour, for example by adding in mechanisms to jiggle the pivot in various ways, driving the

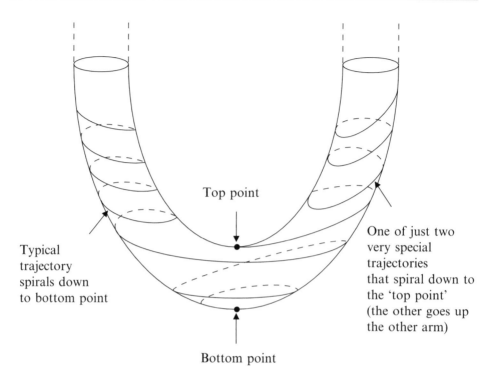

Top point

Typical
trajectory
spirals down
to bottom point

One of just two
very special
trajectories
that spiral down to
the 'top point'
(the other goes up
the other arm)

Bottom point

Figure 2.7   Non-ideal pendulum: phase space as a cylinder.

pendulum (and pushing energy into the system). There are some good tutorial examples of this on the Web.[19]

Let us now examine how these examples illustrate some of the key concepts of dynamical systems theory.

Non-linearity

The equations (17) and (18) describing the system are non-linear. This is what makes the *global* behaviour of the system different from the extrapolation one might make from the *linear approximation* given by the linear version (19) and (20). Globally, there is the u-tube and the pattern of trajectories, whereas for the linearised version the circular orbits would continue out to infinity.

Phase space

We have already seen that the two variables x and y completely determine the state of the system. A *phase space* is a space of points each of which completely determine the state of some system. As the state of the system changes over time, this traces out a path (also known as a *trajectory* or *orbit*) in the phase space.

For either version of the simple pendulum, the phase space is two dimensional. If we were considering a more complicated example of a dynamical system than this, it would be likely to have more than one 'position' variable (like x) and a similar number of 'velocity' variables (like y). Then the phase space, instead of being two dimensional, would be at least four dimensional, and we would have difficulty visualising it (although many mathematicians can handle such spaces with some ease). This shows one reason why it is hard to give a complete visualisable account of more complicated systems which are accessible to the non-mathematician. See also the discussion of statistical mechanics below.

Attractors

An *attractor* is a subset of phase space into which the system 'eventually' settles. The precise (mathematical) definition is quite subtle. For any attractor, there is a neighbourhood, an area of phase space (technically, an open subset) around it, such that any trajectory starting in that area ends up in the attractor. The set of points of phase space whose trajectory ends up in a particular attractor is called the *basin* (or *basin of attraction*) of that attractor.

Attractors can come in an amazing array of shapes and sizes. The attractors in the pendulum examples are as follows:

• The idealised pendulum has no attractors: even for the stable point or the nearly circular orbits there is no (open) basin around them which they 'suck in'. This is connected with the fact that this system is conservative (total energy remains constant), as opposed to dissipative (exchanging energy with its environment).
• For the pendulum with energy drain there is only one attractor, and that is the stable equilibrium point at the bottom of the u-tube. The basin of this attractor consists of the whole u-tube excluding the three orbits of types (b′) and (c′) in the description above (that is, the two orbits that end up just in the unstable equilibrium point, together with that point itself).

The point of stable equilibrium (d′) is a *point attractor*; the other simple type of attractor is a *periodic orbit attractor*. This is a loop like the trajectories of types (a) or (c) in the idealised pendulum (but note that as above these are not themselves attractors). Periodic orbit attractors suck in neighbouring points of phase space, and then the system shows identically repeating behaviour (like the swinging of the idealised pendulum).

For a more complex system the attractors can be extremely 'strange'. There are famous examples in the Lorenz attractor[20] (see p. 6) and the attractors found in other chaotic systems, which are frequently fractal sets of finite fractal dimension[21] (see below for more on fractals). In these cases, it is very common to find that an attractor cannot be given any simple description or explanation: those who try to apply this concept simplistically to complex adaptive systems should beware of this.[22]

Structural stability

When the system of the idealised pendulum was altered slightly, by incorporating an energy drain (even a very small one), the global dynamics of the system, such as the pattern of trajectories, altered greatly, indeed *qualitatively*, in a sense which can be made mathematically precise.[23] This indicates that the idealised pendulum system is not *structurally stable*: a small change in the system produces a dramatic effect. In contrast, the pendulum-with-energy-drain is *structurally stable*: if we alter the system slightly (for example, increase or decrease the rate of energy drain), the qualitative features of the trajectories remain the same.

Open and closed systems, conservative and dissipative systems

It may have seemed strange that the idealised pendulum system had no attractors. It is a *conservative* system, conserving energy. In contrast, the more realistic energy-draining pendulum exchanges energy with its environment: technically it is a *dissipative* system. It is this latter type that shows the more interesting dynamic features. Complex adaptive systems exchange energy or information with their environment, and tend to have complicated attractors.

Emergence and emergent properties

To bring out one further key concept, we need to examine another example of a kind of dynamical system: that dealt with in *statistical mechanics*.

Statistical mechanics concerns itself with substances like gases. Think of a certain mass of gas like air or nitrogen contained in a rigid container, or in a more open situation. The gas is made up of a very large number (call it N) of molecules, each of which is a small particle whose position and velocity can be defined by six coordinate variables (three giving the position in three-dimensional space, three more giving the components of the velocity). The phase space of the total system (the gas in the container) is the 6N-dimensional space with six coordinates for each of the N particles. Take a deep breath – that is a *very* large dimensional space.

The ideas and methods of dynamical systems theory nevertheless apply to this phase space, and so therefore do the concepts, like trajectories and attractors. Additionally, we can easily perceive in this case *emergent properties*.

For gases, the (numerical) properties *temperature*, *pressure* and *entropy* emerge as important ways of describing the system: for example, temperature is a statistical average of the speed of the molecules. These are *emergent* properties: no individual particle has a temperature or a pressure, but the ensemble or system does.

When we consider more general systems like complex adaptive systems, the analogy or metaphor is with dynamical systems as described here. The complex adaptive system is assumed to have a (probably very large) set of variables, which give a complete description of it. These reside in a phase space, and some rules, generally unknown but almost certainly non-linear, define how the system evolves with time. The concepts of trajectories, attractors and emergence may well apply. For example, if we think of the economy (of a region, a country or the world) as a complex adaptive system made up of many interacting actors, the concepts of interest rates, inflation and growth rates emerge.

Fractals and the Mandelbrot set

This section gives a very brief account of fractals, and some references, and concludes with a short description of the 'granddaddy' fractal set, the Mandelbrot set.

A fractal is a mathematical object that can be viewed at a number of different scales (or magnifications) and which 'looks the same' at every scale.[24] This property is known as *self-similarity*. As with many mathematical concepts and objects, examples occur in nature that approximately fit the mathematical form of a fractal. For example, many leaves (like those of some ferns) are composed of leaflets, each of which looks grossly like the whole leaf, and so the leaflet is composed of sub-leaflets, and so on. A natural coastline is another example. If viewed from the air, a coastline appears somewhat wiggly, with inlets, bays, headlands, promontories and so on. From any cliff top, similar patterns are seen at a higher magnification. Down on a beach, the water's edge (at any one time) appears somewhat similar, with indentations and outcrops. Down at the level of individual groups of pebbles and sand grains, 'wiggliness' is still evident, as elaborate as was seen from the air.

Several books examine natural and abstract fractals, often with dazzling pictures.[25]

Fractals are important in dynamical systems theory. Important orbits (and some attractors) have a fractal structure[26]. This can be surprising, and possibly disturbing, since their structure can be extremely complicated ('strange attractors') despite the sometimes apparent simplicity of the dynamical system.

A notable feature of fractals is that they often have in a suitable sense, a fractional dimension.[27] In the coastline example above, one might expect a coastline to be of dimension 1 (a line, albeit a wiggly one). The fact that the coastline 'spreads out' into a second dimension at all levels of magnification shows that it can be said to have a dimension strictly between 1 and 2. This 'Hausdorff dimension' can be given a mathematically precise definition[28] and estimated for real coastlines, typically giving a value around 1.25.[29] One of the most remarkable fractals is the Mandelbrot set, whose definition is given in Box 2.1.

Box 2.1   The Mandelbrot set

If z is a complex variable and c a complex number, the transformation

$$f: \quad z \mapsto z^2 + c \tag{A}$$

maps the complex plane to itself. If we start with a particular complex number, say $z = 0$, we can apply f repeatedly, computing

$$f(z), \ f^2(z) = f(f(z)), \ f^3(z) = f(f(f(z))), \ldots$$

The connection between the initial z and let us say $f^{50}(z)$ is highly non-linear. In fact, for a particular c, only two cases can occur:

$$\text{either } |f^n(0)| \text{ stays bounded as } n \to \infty \tag{B}$$

$$\text{or } |f^n(0)| \to \infty \quad \text{as } n \to \infty \tag{C}$$

(Here $|z|$ is the absolute value of the complex number z.) If c satisfies (B), then we say that c belongs to the Mandelbrot set, a fractal subset of the complex numbers with some remarkable properties.[30]

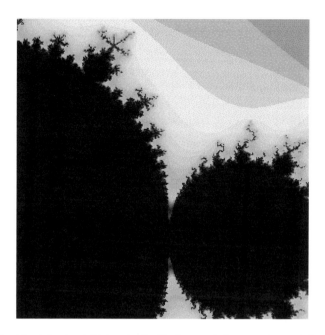

Figure 2.8 The Mandelbrot set. Points in the black areas belong to the set. The boundary between points inside and outside the set has fractal structure.

Chaos and Lyapunov exponents

Chaos is a much-discussed phenomenon in dynamical systems, whereby some orbits show apparently random ('chaotic') behaviour. This is 'abundant in nature',[31] and can be seen in, for example, the case of predator–prey models or the behaviour of epidemics, both of which can be modelled initially and simplistically by the logistic equation.[32]

There are many tools for examining specific examples of chaos.[33] One that is widely used is the concept of *Lyapunov exponents*.[34] This is a relatively difficult mathematical concept, although there is a variety of software that can perform relevant calculations.[35]

Here is a quick outline of two approaches to understanding Lyapunov exponents.

1 The simpler approach looks directly at the way in which nearby points diverge, in the neighbourhood of a point in the phase space of a dynamical system, and constructs a measure of the rate at which this divergence happens.[36] A positive, rather than negative, Lyapunov exponent is a key feature of chaos, because it indicates rapidly growing divergence, and it provides a measure through which chaotic behaviour may be recognised and distinguished both from random noise and from periodicity.

This relatively simple approach glosses over the fact that there are many Lyapunov exponents at any given point, and over an understanding of the corresponding 'principal directions'. It does, however, enable one to talk about the 'three phases' (sigmoid curve) of growth of the divergence,[36] and links well to patterns of chaos in one dimension, as for example in the logistic map.

2 A more complete approach is significantly more technical.[37] It starts with an isolated periodic point x of an orbit (in phase space) of a dynamical system. Using a so-called Poincaré section through x, it produces a linear map from the tangent space at x to itself. This can be represented by a matrix and in a suitable set of axes has a near-diagonal form, which give a set of eigenvalues and corresponding principal directions. The eigenvalues are the Lyapunov exponents at x, and they represent the rate of growth in the divergence of nearby points in the neighbourhood of x. In other words, depending on the 'direction of progress' away from x, the growth of the divergence can be at different rates.

Positive Lyapunov exponents are a key feature of chaos, because they indicate rapidly growing divergence, such as may occur for example with unpredictability in the trajectories evolving from nearby initial conditions.

Conclusion

This chapter has tried to provide a description of the theory on which complexity principles are based. We have seen that terms such as *'non-linearity'* and *'chaos'* have precise mathematical meanings, as well as less formal usages. We have seen that within complex systems, linear approximations are often workable at a local level, but are liable to fail when applied globally to the whole system, which may have emergent properties not reducible to individual components. And we have seen how fractals, a class of geometrical objects that display self-similarity at all scales, represent the dynamics of chaotic behaviour, and are not only amenable to computer simulation, but increasingly recognised in nature.

These expanding fields of study can only be touched on in a single chapter, but this rapid exposition can be followed up through the many references provided.

References

1 See for example http://mathworld.wolfram.com/AffineTransformation.html (accessed 9 November 2003).
2 See for example http://mathworld.wolfram.com/LinearTransformation.html (accessed 9 November 2003).
3 See for example http://mathworld.wolfram.com/LogisticEquation.html (accessed 9 January 2004) and the extended discussion in Chapter 5 of Sweeney K, Griffiths F (eds) (2002) *Complexity and Healthcare: an introduction*, pp. 77–80. Radcliffe Medical Press, Oxford.
4 See www.google.com/search?q = introduction + cryptography or www.google.com/search?q = plaintext + ciphertext or www.faqs.org/faqs/cryptography-faq/ (accessed 9 November 2003).
5 Landshoff P, Metherell A, Rees G (1997) *Essential Quantum Physics* (Chapter 7). Cambridge University Press, Cambridge.

6 Katok A, Hasselblatt B (1995) *Introduction to the Modern Theory of Dynamical Systems*. Cambridge University Press, Cambridge.

7 See for example www.ma.man.ac.uk/~mp/book.html (accessed 9 November 2003) or try www.google.com/search?q = dynamical + systems + theory

8 www.complexityprimarycare.org/glossary.htm (accessed 9 November 2003).

9 Cilliers P (1998) *Complexity and Postmodernism*. Routledge, London.

10 Cilliers P (1998) *Complexity and Postmodernism*. Routledge, London, p. 95.

11 Cilliers P (1998) *Complexity and Postmodernism*. Routledge, London, p. 120.

12 Cilliers P (1998) *Complexity and Postmodernism*. Routledge, London, p. 124.

13 Cilliers P (1998) *Complexity and Postmodernism*. Routledge, London, p. 4.

14 Holland JH (1998) *Emergence*. Addison-Wesley, Boston, MA, pp. 121–2.

15 Nicholis G (1995) *Introduction to Nonlinear Science*. Cambridge University Press, Cambridge, p. 1.

16 See for example http://mathworld.wolfram.com/ContinuousFunction.html (accessed 9 November 2003).

17 See for example Thom R (1993) *Structural Stability and Morphogenesis*. Perseus Publishing, New York, or Katok A, Hasselblatt B (1995) *Introduction to the Modern Theory of Dynamical Systems*, pp. 69–70. Cambridge University Press, Cambridge, or http://mathworld.wolfram.com/StructurallyStable.html (accessed 9 November 2003).

18 See for example www.ma.man.ac.uk/~mp/book.html (accessed 9 November 2003) or try www.google.com/search?q = dynamical + systems + theory

19 See for example The Pendulum Lab: http://monet.physik.unibas.ch//~elmer/pendulum/ (accessed 9 November 2003) and especially http://monet.physik.unibas.ch//~elmer/pendulum/bterm.htm (accessed 9 November 2003); and http://mcasco.com/pend1.html (accessed 9 November 2003).

20 www.sat.t.u-tokyo.ac.jp/~hideyuki/java/Attract.html (accessed 9 November 2003).

21 Nicolis G (1995) *Introduction to Non-linear Science*. Cambridge University Press, Cambridge, p. 222.

22 Compare Kauffman SA (1993) *The Origins of Order*. Oxford University Press, Oxford, pp. 178–9.

23 See for example Katok A, Hasselblatt B (1995) *Introduction to the Modern Theory of Dynamical Systems*. Cambridge University Press, Cambridge, pp. 68–70.

24 http://mathworld.wolfram.com/Fractal.html (accessed 9 November 2003).

25 For example Mandelbrot BB (1982) *The Fractal Geometry of Nature*. WH Freeman, New York, or Barnsley MF (2000) *Fractals Everywhere*. Morgan Kaufmann, San Francisco, or Peitgen HO (1996) *The Beauty of Fractals*. Springer Verlag, New York.

26 Nicolis G (1995) *Introduction to Non-linear Science*. Cambridge University Press, Cambridge, pp. 55–8 and p. 222, or Peitgen HO, Saupe D (eds) (1988) *The Science of Fractal Images*. Springer Verlag, New York, pp. 137–67.

27 http://mathworld.wolfram.com/FractalDimension.html (accessed 9 November 2003).

28 http://polymer.bu.edu/ogaf/html/chp2.htm (accessed 9 November 2003).

29 http://midwoodscience.org/elert/chaos/maine/ (accessed 9 November 2003).

30   See www.google.com/search?q = Mandelbrot + set, for example http://math world.wolfram.com/MandelbrotSet.html or www.mindspring.com/~chroma/ mandelbrot.html or www.olympus.net/personal/dewey/mandelbrot.html or www.math.utah.edu/~alfeld/math/mandelbrot/mandelbrot.html (all accessed 9 November 2003).

31   Nicolis G (1995) *Introduction to Non-linear Science.* Cambridge University Press, Cambridge, p. 173.

32   Sweeney K, Griffiths F (eds) (2002) *Complexity and Healthcare: an introduction.* Radcliffe Medical Press, Oxford, pp. 77–80.

33   Nicolis G (1995) *Introduction to Non-linear Science.* Cambridge University Press, Cambridge, pp. 188–227, or Baker GL, Gollub JP (1996) *Chaotic Dynamics: an introduction.* Cambridge University Press, Cambridge.

34   http://hypertextbook.com/chaos/43.shtml or http://monet.physik.unibas. ch/~elmer/pendulum/lyapexp.htm or http://mathworld.wolfram.com/Lya punovCharacteristicExponent.html (all accessed 9 November 2003).

35   See www.google.com/search?q = lyapunov + exponent + software, for example http://sprott.physics.wisc.edu/chaostsa/ (Chapter 5, accessed 9 November 2003).

36   http://hypertextbook.com/chaos/43.shtml and Nicolis G (1995) *Introduction to Non-linear Science*, Cambridge University Press, Cambridge, pp. 207–10; note the remark on p. 208: 'this view is ... oversimplified'.

37   Katok A, Hasselblatt B (1995) *Introduction to the Modern Theory of Dynamical Systems.* Cambridge University Press, Cambridge, pp. 662–78.

PART TWO

Applying complexity in clinical scenarios

CHAPTER 3

Complexity and the consultation

Andrew Innes

Introduction

The consultation is the central act of medicine. It is what clinicians do and what patients experience as the first part of any clinical episode. Given its significance it is not surprising that it has been extensively studied and researched. This chapter describes in outline how our understanding of the consultation has developed within existing models and then moves on to explore the contribution complexity theory has to make. A model of the consultation as a complex adaptive system is proposed and theoretical aspects of complexity theory are linked to the consultation. The insights offered by such a theoretical approach are then discussed.

Existing consultation models

Many different academic disciplines have brought their own perspective to bear on what happens in consultations between doctors and patients. Medical models of the consultation are doctor-centred, with diagnosis and disease at their core. The purpose of the consultation is to elicit the presence and nature of disease so that it can be treated. This is accomplished through a systematic process of questioning and examination with further investigations arranged as deemed necessary. The medical model of the consultation can therefore be seen as a product of the modernist scientific paradigm where the doctor is viewed as an objective scientific observer. Moreover, this observation is held to be external to the patient's world. Subject—object dualism lies at the core of this model. Cause and effect are seen to be tightly linked and disease is a discrete and identifiable agent. While this model has been very successful in confronting many of the major diseases of the past 200 years it seems inadequate at a number of levels. From the perspective of the patients it seems to ignore their individuality as a factor in the development of disease and also in its management. Furthermore, the complex interactions between individual, disease and society are filtered out. From the doctor's perspective, the capacity for the doctor to be affected by the consultation is not identified. Assumptions, too, are made about the nature of disease as being discrete and identifiable, whereas in fact the disease is but one component of the problems experienced by a patient with an illness.

Sociologists approach the consultation from an entirely different perspective.[1-3] Traditionally, they have been interested in the nature of the interactions between doctors and patients as groups, rather than at the level of individuals. For sociologists, values and norms underpin social action and so they seek to understand those values and norms that relate to medical consultations. They also identify roles as important in promoting and maintaining behaviour. The roles of doctor and patient are seen as clearly identifiable entities each needing to be learned. Anthropologists extend this analysis to consider illness and health-seeking behaviour across cultures.[4,5] Psychological and psychoanalytical models have offered different perspectives.[6–11]

By the late 1970s there was an increasingly held view that illness was the result of the interaction of biological, social and psychological factors, and it was Engel[12] who first proposed this as a model for understanding health and ill health. From this position he then suggested a new model, the bio-psycho-social model, as the basis for the interaction between patients and healthcare professionals.[13,14] Engel's proposal was an important step forward, but while it provided a welcome opportunity to describe health and the interaction of patients and professionals, it offered no insights into the dynamics of that interaction. It allows us to understand that biological, social and psychological factors contribute to health, but provides no understanding of the relative effects of each component.

More recently, general practitioners (GPs) have developed their own models of the consultation in the context of consultation skills training.[15,16] While these have been useful in the training of GPs, they have provided little in terms of understanding how consultations really work.

Each of these models brings a different and useful perspective to bear on our understanding of the consultation, but their utility is reduced by the bounded nature of disciplinary thinking on which they are based, be it sociological, psychological or medical. Furthermore they offer only limited insights into the dynamics operating in consultations.

Complexity theory

In the past few years, there has been a developing interest in complexity theory as a way of understanding what happens in health and healthcare.[17–21] Complexity theory can be seen as a development of systems thinking informed by chaos theory and a family of theories which include dissipative structures, complex adaptive systems and, most recently, complex responsive processes.[22–24] Systems thinking was itself born in the 1950s with the creation of the Society for General Systems Research.[25] The original aims of systems thinking are expressed in Box 3.1.

Box 3.1 The aims of the Society for General Systems Research

- To investigate the isomorphy of concepts, laws and models in various fields and to help in useful transfers from one field to another.
- To encourage the development of adequate theoretical models in fields which lack them.
- To eliminate the duplication of theoretical efforts in different fields.
- To promote the unity of science through improving communication between specialists.

Seen in this light, complexity theory, perhaps the best contender currently for a general systems theory, offers the possibility of a coherent link between the various strands of thinking about the consultation. Indeed, Dean has suggested that complexity completes our understanding of Engel's bio-psycho-social model by providing an explanation of the interaction between the parts of the model.[26]

Complexity and the consultation

Although complexity theory offers a framework for understanding all consultations, this understanding is not always helpful or necessary. Some consultations are concerned with simple matters where actions and intended outcomes are easily agreed between clinicians and patients. Figure 3.1 shows a useful framework for considering this.[24,27]

Along one axis we move from being close to certainty to being far from certainty, while the other similarly describes agreement. At a point close to certainty and close to agreement, cause and effect relationships are most clearly seen by both doctor and patient and a consensus on action is most easily achieved. A patient with an inguinal hernia who wants surgical treatment would be an example. As we move further away from agreement and yet certainty is relatively preserved, we move into an area where political decision making becomes more

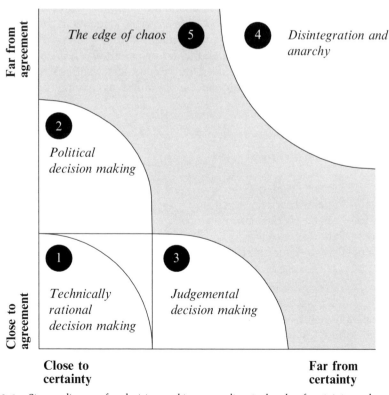

Figure 3.1   Stacey diagram for decision making according to levels of certainty and agreement.

important. Here the clinical evidence may be clear but consensus is difficult to achieve. This can be seen in the current debate in the UK about the safety of MMR vaccination. Moving in the other direction, agreement remains strong but the evidence is less clear. In this zone, decision making becomes more a matter of judgement. Aspects of palliative care would fit this zone. As we move further towards a point far from certainty and far from agreement, the consultation may break down. In this anarchic region, there is neither certainty nor agreement and no progress can be made. Between the zone of technically rational decisions and anarchy, the consultation may be complex. This is where much of the clinical activity of general practice takes place. Links between cause and effect are unclear and there is uncertainty about the way forward. Undifferentiated problems are presented and symptoms are frequently vague. These problems are the most diffi-cult to help but can also be the most rewarding. Fatigue, chronic pain, somatisa-tion and a range of mental health disorders occupy this zone, but any clinical problem might at some time come to rest here either as a result of circumstances or its evolution.

Diversity and agency in the consultation

Diversity is the key to understanding complex adaptive systems. It can be seen at many levels within the consultation. Diversity is the key to innovation and long-term viability. It equates in biological and business systems with success. It can first be seen at the level of agency within the consultation. Agents are the basic components of a complex adaptive system and a number of them can be identified within the consultation. Doctors and patients are clearly agents in their own rights but a nurse, GP registrar or medical student might also be present. Patients might also be accompanied by a partner, friend, child or parent. Even if unaccompanied, patients attend consultations influenced by friends and relatives. Helman[28] has suggested five clinical triads that can be regarded as having agency within consultations (Box 3.2).

Box 3.2   Helman's clinical triads

1   Doctor–Patient–Manager
2   Doctor–Patient–Lawyer
3   Doctor–Patient–Statistician
4   Doctor–Patient–Journalist
5   Doctor–Patient–Computer

The first triad describes the influence of management on the consultation. Doctors have increasingly had to come to terms with more managed healthcare in the UK. Targets and contract influences have increased and are likely to continue to do so. Furthermore, GPs are moving more towards being part of the larger organisational culture of primary care trusts, which is likely to further enhance the sense of mana-gerial influence. The influence of the lawyer hovering in the background is inevit-able with an increasing number of complaints and increased litigation. The impact of this trend has been to investigate further, seeking corroborative data wherever possible, and to increase referral rates. High-profile cases have undermined both public and professional confidence in the nature of the doctor–patient relationship. The statistician comes to the consultation in two ways. First, we live in an age of measurement of targets and rates of everything from prescribing to cervical cytology. Our second encounter with the statistician comes in the form of evidence-based medicine. Here, doctors struggle to evaluate essentially population-based and largely secondary care-oriented research in the context of helping individual patients. The role of the media in consultations is familiar to all and is one of the 'cues to action' in Rosenstock's health belief model.[7] Although largely considered to be beneficial, there have been concerns that media influences have raised patient expectations to unrealistic heights at times and have also created distorted ideas about the nature of risk.

Most general practices have been computerised[29] and indeed many are now paperless.[30] Computers have become an entirely indispensible part of modern general practice capable of delivering the prizes of high-quality notes, data and audit, and yet they influence the consultation[31] in many ways, some of which are less subtle than others. They compete for eye contact and it has even been suggested that they reinforce a mechanical, non-human view of the self.[32] Wider socio-cultural influences, whether religious, social or economic, can also act as agents.

Stacey describes narrative themes as having agency within what he prefers to describe as a complex responsive process.[24] The emphasis on narrative is important because it underlines the richness of an individual's story and implores us to consider the dangers inherent in reducing that story to the level of a technical description. Stacey also describes organising themes as experiences that mould the way we are and the way we respond, and these too can act as agents. An example of an organising theme from general practice might be the experience of patients who seek advice about a sore throat and are prescribed an antibiotic. When those patients next experience similar symptoms they might quite reasonably assume that the appropriate course of action is to go back to their doctor, believing that they need more antibiotics.

Free-flowing conversation is a process by which the space of possibilities can be explored.[24] Where conversation is constrained in consultations, then important information and perspectives cannot emerge. Imperfections in communication akin to the mistakes and repairs identified and explicated by conversation analysis[33,34] may act as agents in the consultation, changing its direction. The skills required here are for the doctor to enable free-flowing conversation within the consultation and to remain sensitive to the insights that imperfections in communication may throw up.

A variety of contextual agents also act in the consultation. The physical environment of the waiting room and then the consulting room exert their own influences, as does the organisation of the practice. Time within any one consultation is constrained and this constraint can act as an agent in its own right, significantly affecting what happens.

Co-evolution in consultations

Complex adaptive systems change over time and the agents within them co-evolve, each agent changing in response to the changing context, which includes changes in the other agents in the system. Doctors and patients arrive at a consultation with a prior history and often base management on symptoms rather than diagnosis, as a clinical picture emerges. As symptoms change so does the management. Relationships with patients and perspectives on their problems also emerge over time; both are changed by their interaction and new perspectives emerge.

Distributed control

Control within a complex adaptive system is *distributed,* with outcomes emerging from a process of self-organisation rather than being the result of design or external control. Distributed control is itself intimately bound up with the concept of simple rules.[35–37] Very complex behaviour such as flocking birds has been explained in terms of simple rules.[38] Another way of considering the variety created by a limited set of simple rules is to consider how different any two games of soccer are, even between the same two teams. Rules have been discussed in relation to a variety of aspects of medical practice in the past. For example, rules have been proposed as the basis for protecting patients. Gorovitz and MacIntyre[39] identified that:

> A profession concerned to minimise malpractice should then specify as well as possible the canons of good practice.

In other words, at the level of patient safety, rules are important and transgression of these rules or 'deontological offence' is the essence of malpractice. However, rules in complex systems are not deterministic and what emerges is not necessarily predictable. It is perhaps this aspect of complexity that offers the most radical and controversial view of the consultation, in that the traditional idea of the locus of control being the doctor is rejected and replaced by the understanding of control based on the relationships between agents and influences acting within the consultation.

So what sort of rules might operate in the consultation? Certainly there are social rules or conventions that govern the interaction of doctors and patients in the sociological sense of roles. Related to these are the conversational rules picked up in the study of conversation.[33] Ethical rules can also be seen to be in play and supporting the role of 'doctor'. The GMC's publication *Good Medical Practice,*[40] on the other hand, identifies 13 different rules governing clinical care. Returning to Pendleton[15] and Neighbour,[16] they essentially offer a rule-based system for the conduct of consultations.

A further property of distributed control is that emergence is essentially unpredictable, which once again challenges deeply held ideas and models of what medical consultations should generate. Both doctors and their patients like to feel that the medical process that they embark upon during the consultation is safe and predictable, which complexity theory undermines. And yet, if we look closely at a number of aspects of the consultation, the complexity model with its inherent uncertainty and unpredictability does indeed seem to fit better with the experience and reality of medical practice.

Non-linearity

In a complex system, the size of any input does not correlate with its output in a linear or predictable manner. A very small action or observation may entirely transform the assessment and management of a patient's problem. Similarly, a large input may have very little effect. The principle consequence of non-linearity is that it creates an environment that permits perpetual novelty and creativity. Like distributed control, it is also a mechanism by which uncertainty is created. Clinicians see non-linearity in their work every day. Chance remarks, minor observations and 'minor' clinical data such as a single mildly abnormal or even normal laboratory result might send consultations off in very different directions. For example, a patient may present with a history of chest pain that would fit the characteristics of cardiac pain and yet the clinician might detect subtle non-verbal clues suggestive of depression that is at the root of the patient's physical symptoms.

Consultation patterns and creativity

Even though consultations are constrained and some similarities can be expected because of the interactions of the individual agents, each consultation is different. This is true even when the clinician is the same. Consider the doctor reviewing a hypertensive patient. Talk centres on symptoms, medication problems and attention to cardiovascular risk analysis. The process is doctor-led and frequently follows a pattern of talk and activity used with many patients, and also repeatedly with an individual patient over time. The nature of this consultation may inhibit the emergence of new information if patterns of talk and action are predictable and novelty stifled or ignored. In contrast, a consultation characterised by the facilitation of free-flowing conversation allows the expression of novelty and creativity and perhaps a glimpse of new and surprising insights that may lead the consultation into completely new areas. This fits with our understanding of complex adaptive systems as being fairly robust and stable, and yet dynamic with the capacity for dramatic change. A stable pattern of consultation may be appropriate, but there are times in general practice when we need to think more creatively when trying to work out why we are unable to effect a clearly beneficial change in a patient's behaviour or understand their current pattern of behaviour.

Consultations at the edge of chaos

Complex adaptive systems thrive in areas of bounded instability, and Kauffman suggests that complex systems move to the edge of chaos to solve problems.[36,37] The consultation in this zone will move from safe, familiar territory to less familiar patterns of talk and action. Consultations might move into this zone either because the clinician or patient moves them there deliberately in an attempt to destabilise a particular consultation pattern, or by a process of co-evolution. With this shift, the opportunity to gain new insights and create new opportunities for change arises. Novelty and creativity are the hallmarks of this area. However, both in terms of the relationship between the doctor and patient and any intervention arising from the consultation, consulting at the edge of chaos implies risk. This risk might be to the doctor–patient relationship or may relate to the unpredictable possibilities arising from a clinical intervention such as the prescription of medication or the use of a psychological therapy.

Consider the following case:

Case study

A 55-year-old taxi driver with a past history of angina presented to his GP with chest pain. He had not had any chest pain since coronary artery intervention 4 years earlier. His description of his chest pain was vague and his GP, who knew him well and considered his relationship with the patient to be good, felt increasingly frustrated by his inability to work out whether or not his symptoms represented a re-emergence of his angina. Eventually the GP overtly challenged the patient and asked him if he was being 'deliberately obtuse' in his vague responses. The patient looked completely shocked by this departure from any of the 'rules' that had determined the basis of their previous interactions and a brief period of silence ensued. After this the patient described his concerns and fears about the possible significance of his symptoms. What might they mean for his health and mortality and what were the implications for his job?

In this example the usual patterns of interaction between the doctor and patient, which were comfortable for both of them, were inhibiting expression of the real problem. By challenging the patient, the consultation moved from its position of stability towards the edge of chaos, where new insights were gained but a risk was taken with the relationship between doctor and patient.

Chaos

Intuitively, of course, all of those of us who consult will have our own idea of what marks a consultation as chaotic. A chaotic system in a theoretical sense, however, conveys fairly specific meaning. Chaotic behaviour, despite its outward impression, is not random. It is unpredictable but to an extent deterministic. The level of determinism, however, is such that it is exquisitely sensitive to initial conditions, and very small differences in these initial conditions can make an enormous difference or no difference. As Byrne says,[41] chaos is the 'precursor of order and not its antithesis'. So within a chaotic system, islands of linearity and coherence exist. Set in the context of a consultation, the overall pattern would be that the traditional sequence and patterns of the progress of the consultation are lost and the outcomes become difficult to predict. Risk is implied because problems are not identified and/or not dealt with. And yet within this chaotic dynamic, recognisable patterns do exist, such as a sequence of clear history from a patient or a question or part of a physical examination from a doctor. The links, however, are not made and the consultation is unsafe. Such a framework may offer interesting insights into a doctor's poor performance in a consultation.

Insights from complexity theory

The consultation can be described as a complex adaptive system. As such, clinical consultations are seen as complex responsive processes where meaning emerges often unpredictably from the interaction between the patient and the clinician. The role of the clinician therefore becomes one of an enquiring participant who seeks to influence change in a patient's condition. Such a view offers a number of helpful insights.

The single most important advantage of understanding the consultation as a complex adaptive system is that it takes into account uncertainty and unpredictability. For too long the medical process has been presented as one based on predictability and certainty supported by the myth of physician supremacy and the power of modern medicine. The 'necessary fallibility'[39] that arises from the complexity of individuals and health has been largely ignored. This places an unrealistic pressure on the doctor to find successful solutions to all problems and denies the patient the opportunity to share and understand the uncertain reality of illness and healthcare. Complexity theory reveals the reality of uncertainty within medicine and the emergent unpredictability of what happens in consultations, easing the tension felt by clinicians. It acknowledges the need for the doctor to be able to display what Stacey describes as 'good-enough holding of anxiety'.[24] The duty of the doctor here is to be aware of the levels of uncertainty operating in a particular case and work with them in a way that is as safe as can be reasonably possible. From the perspective of patients, the doctor's ability to tolerate uncertainty will have a major impact on their experience of healthcare. Where the ability to work with uncertainty is reduced, a patient may be exposed to prolonged referral and investigation processes that are likely to provoke and maintain anxiety in situations where discovery of significant and remedial pathology is highly unlikely. Beyond this, the doctor working either with physical or psychological illness has a role to play in 'holding' the anxiety a patient feels as they work through a particular health problem. Friedman[42] describes this role in the context of family therapy as that of a caretaker, where the caretaker's and patient's capacity to tolerate anxiety mutually influence each other.

Complexity also identifies the individual as being a group member, and while this is familiar within most models of the consultation, it is central to complexity theory. An individual patient is a complex adaptive system nested within other complex adaptive systems, as is the doctor. An important consequence of this is that subject/object dualism is denied and the doctor cannot be seen as an objective external observer as suggested by traditional medical models of the doctor–patient interaction. The actions and communication of doctors and patients within a consultation each have an impact on the other becoming the agents of a complex system with intrinsic emergent unpredictability.

If a systemic interpretation of complexity theory is adopted then it also offers a strategic framework for considering the consultation and reminds us of the possibilities of systemic intervention. Bearing in mind the Stacey matrix, it is possible for doctors to be aware of the consultation territory in which they find themselves and adopt an appropriate strategy. However, when consultations become stuck then manoeuvring towards the edge of chaos offers new opportunities to gain helpful insights, as in the case example above. These insights might, however, disclose possible interventions in the wider context of the patient as an embedded system.

Conclusions

Complexity theory and its principles resonate with the experience of the practice of medicine, particularly in the undifferentiated environment of primary care. It offers a coherent theoretical framework for understanding consultations and their emergent outcomes. More than this, however, it offers new insights that increase our understanding of consultations. Returning to the aims of systems thinking, complexity theory also offers the possibility of developing a language that doctors, patients and society at large can share, which provides a meaningful understanding of uncertainty and unpredictability in healthcare.

Acknowledgements

I would like to thank Professor Peter Campion and Dr Frances Griffiths for their help and support in the development of this work.

References

1   Mechanic D (1962) The concept of illness behaviour. *Journal of Chronic Disease*. **15**: 189–94.
2   Tuckett D (1976) *An Introduction to Medical Sociology*. Tavistock, London.
3   Boreham P, Gibson D (1978) The informative process in private medical consultations: a preliminary investigation. *Social Science*. **12**: 409–16.
4   Kleinman A (1980) *Patients and Healers in the Context of Culture*. University of California, Berkeley.
5   Helman C (1981) Diseases versus illness in general practice. *BJGP*. **31**: 548–52.
6   Balint M (1968) *The Doctor, His Patient and the Illness* (2e). Pitman, London.
7   Rosenstock I (1966) Why patients use health services. *Millbank Memorial Fund Quarterly*. **44**: 94–127.
8   Berne E (1964) *Games People Play*. Penguin, Harmondsworth.
9   Rotter J (1966) Generalized expectancies for internal vs. external control of reinforcement. *Psychol Monogr*. **80**(609).
10 Byrne P, Heath C (1980) Practitioners' use of non verbal behaviour in real consultations. *BJGP*. **30**: 327–31.
11 Byrne P, Long B (1976) *Doctors Talking to Patients*. HMSO, London.
12 Engel G (1977) The need for a new medical model: a challenge for biomedicine. *Science*. **196**: 129–36.
13 Engel G (1978) The biopsychosocial model and the education of health professionals. *Annals of the New York Academy of Sciences*. **310**: 169–81.
14 Engel G (1980) The clinical application of the biopsychosocial model. *American Journal of Psychiatry*. **137**: 535–44.
15 Pendleton D, Schofield T, Tate P, Havelock P (1984) *The Consultation: an approach to learning and teaching*. Oxford University Press, Oxford.
16 Neighbour R (1999) *The Inner Consultation: how to develop an effective and intuitive consulting style*. Petroc Press, Newbury.
17 Griffiths F, Byrne D (1998) General practice and the new science emerging from the theories of 'chaos' and complexity. *BJGP*. **48**: 1697–99.

18   Plsek P, Greenhalgh T (2001) The challenge of complexity in health care. *BMJ*. **323**: 625–8.

19   Wilson T, Holt T, Greenhalgh T (2001) Complexity and clinical care. *BMJ*. **323**: 685–8.

20   Plsek P, Wilson T (2001) Complexity, leadership, and management in healthcare organisations. *BMJ*. **323**: 746–9.

21   Fraser S, Greenhalgh T (2001) Coping with complexity: educating for capability. *BMJ*. **323**: 799–803.

22   Prigogine I, Stengers I (1984) *Order Out of Chaos: man's new dialogue with nature*. Bantam, New York.

23   Waldrop M (1992) *Complexity: the emerging science at the edge of order and chaos*. Viking, London.

24   Stacey R (2000) *Strategic Management and Organizational Dynamics* (3e). Financial Times/Prentice Hall, Harlow.

25   Jackson M (2000) *Systems Approaches to Management*. Kluwer/Plenum, New York.

26   Dean A (2001) Complexity and substance misuse. *Addiction Research and Theory*. **9**(1): 19–41.

27   Zimmerman B, Lindberg C, Plsek P (2001) *Edgeware: insights from complexity science for healthcare leaders*. VHA, Irving, TX.

28   Helman C (2002) The culture of general practice. *BJGP*. **52**: 619–20.

29   NHS Executive (1998) *Computerisation in General Practice Survey*. Department of Health, London.

30   Waring T (2000) To what extent are general practices 'paperless' and what are the constraints to them becoming more so? *BJGP*. **50**: 46–7.

31   Muir Gray J (1999) Postmodern medicine. *Lancet*. **354**: 1550–3.

32   Turke S (1984) *The Second Self: computers and the human spirit*. Granada, London.

33   Ten Have P (1999) *Doing Conversational Analysis: a practical guide*. Sage, London.

34   Jefferson G (1987) On exposed and embedded correction in conversation. In: G Button, J Lee (eds) *Talk and Social Interaction*, pp. 86–100. Multilingual Matters, Clevedon, PA.

35   Holland J (1998) *Emergence from Chaos to Order*. Oxford University Press, New York.

36   Kauffman S (1993) *Origins of Order: self-organization and selection in evolution*. Oxford University Press, Oxford.

37   Kauffman S (1995) *At Home in the Universe*. Oxford University Press, New York.

38   Reynolds C (1987) Flocks, herds and schools: a distributed behaviour model. *Computer Graphics*. **21**(4): 25–34.

39   Gorovitz S, MacIntyre A (1976) Toward a theory of medical fallibility. *Journal of Medicine and Philosophy*. **1**(1): 51–71.

40   General Medical Council (2001) *Good Medical Practice*. GMC, London.

41   Byrne D (1998) *Complexity Theory and the Social Sciences* (1e). Routledge, London.

42   Friedman EH (1985) *Generation to Generation: family process in church and synagogue*. Guildford, New York.

CHAPTER 4

Complexity, chaos and cardiology

David C Aron

The practice of cardiology involves understanding the pathophysiology of cardiac diseases and, in order to apply that knowledge effectively, an understanding of the delivery of cardiac healthcare. This understanding spans multiple levels from cell to organ to whole person to healthcare delivery unit, to aggregation of units into healthcare facilities and delivery systems. These systems and subsystems are all open systems in which there is exchange of energy and information across boundaries; these levels communicate with each other and are influenced by other systems as well. Moreover, each of these systems is dynamic.

The multiplicity of interactions within and between systems, the non-linear characteristics of those interactions and their dynamic nature brings to the practice of cardiology a high degree of uncertainty and unpredictability.[1] An individual patient may or may not respond to a specific treatment, even a treatment whose benefit has been well established by randomised controlled trials. Cardiac patients often require urgent intervention; how well the healthcare team communicates during cardiopulmonary resuscitation influences the likelihood of success. Traditional approaches to studying these systems have been reductionist – isolating components to learn more about them.

Complexity and chaos theory offer a different approach that more explicitly recognises interactions, non-linearity and the dynamic nature of systems. Blood pressure, blood flow, heart rate behaviour and heart rate variability are regulated by a series of feedback mechanisms. Similar mechanisms are involved in the operations of a coronary care unit (CCU) as well as all of the levels from individual cells to an entire hospital. Because the mathematics of chaos can be daunting even to those who are not mathematically squeamish, this chapter will provide a non-technical approach to the role of complexity and chaos in cardiology. Readers interested in a more rigorous approach are referred to a number of fine books, papers and websites.[2–8]

'Complexity theory' is not a theory per se, but rather a loose set of concepts, orientations, heuristics and analytic tools.[9,10] Complexity is related to the branch of mathematics known as chaos and chaos theory. Although there are controversies about what chaos is, one useful definition is 'stochastic behavior occurring in a deterministic system'. That is, chaos occurs when a non-random (deterministic) system behaves in an apparently random or chance (stochastic) manner.[3] Chaos theory shows that 'simple' systems can exhibit complex behaviour, while complexity theory shows that 'complex' systems can exhibit simple (emergent) behaviour.

Both involve non-linear phenomena, interactions and change over time, i.e. dynamic behaviour.[3] The concepts can be applied in cardiology from the cell to the bedside. Manson proposed a division of complexity research:

- *deterministic complexity*, which deals with chaos theory and catastrophe theory
- *aggregate complexity*, which deals with how individual elements work in concert to create systems with complex behaviour
- *algorithmic complexity*, which involves mathematical complexity theory and information theory.[11]

Each of these themes applies to cardiology. In this chapter we will focus on the first two.

Deterministic complexity

In a deterministic system, the system is completely characterised. Given the same starting conditions and the same equation, the same results would be produced. However, chaotic behaviour is very sensitive to initial conditions; small differences in values at the start may result in huge differences later on; large differences in values at the start may result in small or no differences later on. Although the future behaviour at a particular future point in time cannot be predicted with certainty, the behaviour of the system as a whole can be described within limits; chaotic systems often appear to nearly (but never quite) repeat themselves, and certainly seem to gravitate to some features (either absolute values or 'trajectories') – attractors. *Fractals* constitute part of the mathematics of chaos.

Fractal patterns in anatomical structures and physiological processes

The term 'fractal' was coined by the mathematician B Mandelbrot and first applied as a geometric/mathematical concept related to chaos.[12–14] In contrast to lines, planes and solids, which have integer dimensions of 1, 2 and 3 respectively, a fractal object is one with parts that resemble smaller copies of the whole over a range of scale. For example, a branching structure (Figure 4.1a), which has a dimension between 1 and 2, somewhere between a line and a plane, illustrates a fractal line. Closer examination at finer resolution reveals subunits, which mimic that of the larger structure. These subunits are composed of even smaller, but geometrically similar subunits. This is the property of *self-similarity*. A fractal object has features over a broad range of sizes. A consequence is that the length of the overall structure depends on the resolution at which the fractal is measured. At higher resolutions, finer features are revealed and the length measured will be longer. The scaling relationship defines how the measured properties depend on the resolution used to make the measurement. This relationship may obey the power law or other mathematical laws. The *fractal dimension* yields a quantitative measure of self-similarity and scaling, indicating how many new subunits are revealed at higher resolutions.

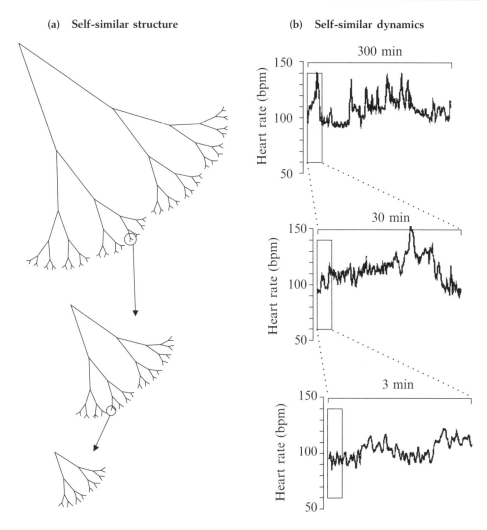

Figure 4.1 (a) Schematic of a tree-like fractal has self-similar branchings such that the small-scale (magnified) structure resembles the large-scale form. (b) A fractal process such as heart rate regulation generates fluctuations on different timescales (temporal 'magnifications') that are statistically self-similar. © *Lancet*. (Adapted with permission from Goldberger AL (1996) Non-linear dynamics for clinicians: chaos theory, fractals, and complexity at the bedside. *Lancet*. **347**: 1312–14.)

Fractals may be purely mathematical structures that exhibit these properties over an infinite range of scales. However, real-world objects may be described as fractals or fractal-like with the self-similarity of fractal geometry over a finite range of scales. Unlike mathematically defined objects, with real-world objects, the parts are not exact copies of the larger parts, but rather statistically similar. The fractal nature of biological systems is readily illustrated in branching patterns of trees. The heart is replete with such branching structures: the coronary arteries and veins, the conduction fibres in the heart (His–Purkinje system) and the fibres binding the valves to the heart wall, among others.[12–14]

There are several implications of fractal structure. First, analogous to the fact that complex fractals can be produced with simple mathematical expressions, biological structures are complex, but are coded by relatively few genes. The genetic information may be relatively simple, but it can produce complex structure and functions through chaotic processes. Second, functionally, the fractal structures of the heart allow for rapid and efficient transport over a complex, spatially distributed system.[13,14] Fractal branching makes available much more surface area for absorption and transfer of oxygen, nutrients and waste products in the coronary circulation and does so in a relatively homogeneous fashion. Similarly, the large surface area of the tracheo-bronchial tree facilitates gas exchange.[15] In a sense, the coronary vessels and the branching tracheo-bronchial tree are fractals with dimensions between 2 and 3, converting a volume of blood in the artery or gas in the trachea (dimension = 3) into something approaching a surface area (dimension = 2) in the capillaries and alveoli.

The cardiac conduction system ensures the efficient transport of electrical signals that regulate the timing of cardiac contraction. The fractal organisation of connective tissue in the aortic valve leaflets relates to the efficient distribution of mechanical forces.[16] The *redundancy* of fractal structures renders them more robust and resistant to injury. For example, the heart can continue to function even after considerable damage to a major coronary artery or the His–Purkinje system. Sapoval suggested that 'the fractal structure of the human circulatory system damps out the hammer blows that our heart generates ... The heart is a very violent pump, and if there were any resonance in blood circulation, you would die.'[17,18] Finally, fractals constitute useful mathematical models that yield insights into normal physiology and pathophysiology. For example, analysis of the fractal dimension of pulmonary blood vessels illustrates differences between the normal and disease states.[19] The fractal dimension is a measure of how many additional blood vessel branches are found as smaller blood vessels are examined. Hypobaric and hyperbaric oxygen are associated with higher pulmonary arterial pressures. Boxt *et al.* determined the fractal dimension of these blood vessels in rats reared in hypoxic, high oxygen and normal environments.[19] They found that the fractal dimension of the blood vessels in the normal lungs was 1.65, while fractal dimension of the blood vessels in the abnormal lungs was 1.53 and 1.43, for hypoxia and hyperbaric oxygen respectively. The blood vessels from lungs of rats reared in these non-physiologic environments had fewer, finer branches than vessels from the normal lungs. In fact, different mechanisms appear to produce fractals with different dimensions. Thus, the fractal dimension of a structure may hint at the underlying mechanism that produced it. For example, the process called diffusion-limited aggregation produces fractals with a fractal dimension of about 1.7. The blood vessels in the retina have a fractal dimension of about 1.7. Thus, it is worthwhile to consider if the growth of these blood vessels was produced by diffusion-limited aggregation. This would mean that the growth of the blood vessels was proportional to the gradient of a diffusible substance, such as oxygen or a growth factor.[8]

The embryologic development of the pulmonary vascular tree can be modelled by fractal branching algorithms and boundaries that change as the embryo develops.[20] Despite the fact that these models are two-dimensional models, they yield remarkably realistic vascular patterns. Blood flow in the heart can also be described in fractal terms.[12] For example, Bassingthwaighte *et al.*, using a radioactive tracer method, assessed blood flow by calculating the relative dispersion (RD), a measure equal to the standard deviation divided by the average of the blood flow measured in a piece of any given weight.[21] In measuring the blood flow in pieces of different weight, they found that RD had the power law scaling relationship, such that RD was proportional to w^{1-d}, where $w =$ weight and $d =$ fractal dimension. Thus, blood flow is heterogeneous and fractal. Regions of the heart vary in their blood flow; some have higher-than-average blood flow while others have lower-than-average blood flow. Moreover, in following a scaling relationship, the pattern of blood flow exhibits self-similarity. Both large and small and still smaller regions vary in their blood flow in similar ways. Similar studies have been performed in a variety of species. In addition to demonstrating the spatial heterogeneity of myocardial blood flow, this approach allows the ready comparison of the fractal dimensions. Interestingly, differences were observed, suggesting functional and morphogenetic differences.[21] Like physical branching structures, blood flow heterogeneity can be fractal only over a limited range.

Fractal analysis provides a geometric framework for the description of apparently irregular patterns, facilitating the characterisation of processes and structures that are not easily represented by the traditional analytic tools.[12,22] Glenny[12] stated:

> Because there cannot possibly be a complete genetic description for the construction of every alveolus and capillary, it seems logical to propose that there are elementary recursive rules to guide their construction. These construction codes are probably not fractal themselves but are likely deterministic rules defining basic elements that are influenced by the environment in which the structure grows. The branching structures of the vascular system and the bronchial tree are such examples, where it is not known whether the branching angles and diameters are determined by the parent branch or by the similar environment in which they are constructed. Although the mechanisms by which these rules operate are speculative, a coding for self-similar structures is clearly the most efficient and appropriate algorithm to explain both the order and complexity of ontogeny. The efficiency of the finalized structures is also of importance to the organism.

Just as the mathematical concept of fractals provides insights into complex anatomic branching structures that lack a characteristic (single) length scale, they also apply to complex physiologic processes, such as heart rate regulation, that lack a single timescale. Fractal processes generate irregular fluctuations across multiple timescales, analogous to scale-invariant objects that have a branching or wrinkly structure across multiple length scales.[23] This can be readily seen in Figure 4.1b, which plots a time series of heart rate fluctuation in three different timescales. Each plot has an irregular appearance and each resembles, although is not identical to, the others – self-similarity. While this method is qualitative, other methods are available that provide a more rigorous representation of the temporal self-similarity of the healthy heartbeat, e.g. wavelet analysis.[23] Such scale-invariance characterises many physiological functions in the heart and elsewhere, from the cellular level to the whole organ, from certain ion channel kinetics to heart rate variability (HRV).

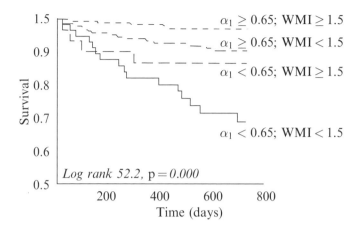

Figure 4.2   Kaplan–Meier survival curves of patients divided into different subgroups according to the short-term scaling exponent α_1 and wall motion index (WMI). The patients were divided into two groups based on their left ventricular systolic function, and the predictive power of the short-term scaling exponent was analysed in each group. Reduced values of α_1 predicted a significantly increased risk of mortality in both groups. A consecutive series of 806 patients were screened in three centres (Gentofte and Glostrup Hospitals, Copenhagen, Denmark, and Oulu University Hospital, Oulu, Finland). © *Excerpta Medica*. (Adapted with permission from Tapanainen J, Thomsen P, Køber L *et al.* (2002) Fractal analysis of heart rate variability and mortality after an acute myocardial infarction. *American Journal of Cardiology*. **90**: 347–52.)

Heart rate variability

The term 'heart rate variability' (HRV) refers to both the oscillation in the interval between consecutive heart beats (R–R intervals) and to the oscillations between consecutive instantaneous heart rates.[24] This variability reflects the complex feedback mechanisms involved in heart rate regulation, in particular autonomic regulation.[25] Blood pressure variability has also been examined.[25] The relevance of HRV to clinical practice has been evident for nearly 40 years.[24] Analysis of HRV has been used to evaluate autonomic regulation of the sinus node in both normal subjects and in patients with a variety of cardiac as well as non-cardiac diseases.[24,26,27] Such analysis has assumed particular importance in the identification of patients at risk for an increased cardiac mortality. Wolf *et al.* demonstrated that patients with low magnitude of short-term HRV have poor prognosis after acute myocardial infarction.[28] These results have been confirmed in a variety of studies using different methods for assessment of HRV.[29] The prognostic value of HRV parameters has also been demonstrated in patients with heart failure.[30] In fact, in the Framingham Heart Study, a large population-based epidemiological study, depressed HRV was associated with an increased incidence of subsequent cardiac events, including angina, myocardial infarction and congestive heart failure, even in subjects apparently free of coronary disease or congestive heart failure at the time of the HRV measurement.[31] Reduction in HRV identifies diabetic autonomic neuropathy, which is associated with a high mortality rate – 50% at 5 years.[23,32–35] There are also age-related changes in HRV, specifically reduction in the magnitude of HRV.

A variety of methods have been used to assess HRV.[24,29] The work of the Task Force of the North American Society of Pacing and Electrophysiology and the

European Society of Cardiology to unify and standardise the methods for measurement of HRV notwithstanding, there is little agreement about what constitutes
the best method or index for clinical or research use.[24,29,36–38] Most commonly,
HRV has been assessed by time domain parameters related to statistical operations
on R–R intervals (means and variance), e.g. average heart rate (HR) and standard
deviation of all normal-to-normal R–R intervals over a specific time period. (It is
obvious that some method needs to be used to deal with premature beats and
related compensatory pauses.) Frequency domain parameters usually assessed by
spectral analysis have also been used. Such parameters have certain advantages,
though their predictive ability has not been that much greater than that of time
domain measures.[13] More recently, non-linear and fractal analytic techniques have
been applied. They are designed to assess the qualitative properties of the signal
rather than the magnitude of variability; the normal heart rate time series exhibits
self-similarity over various time scales (fractal scaling component), which can be
measured using a variety of sophisticated mathematical methods. Other non-linear
measures have been used, e.g. approximate entropy, which measures the regularity
and complexity of time series data by quantifying the likelihood that runs of
patterns that are close remain close on next incremental comparisons.[39] However,
as pointed out by Mäkikallio[29]:

> whether the various nonlinear methods detect nonlinear behavior is an
> important scientific issue, but from the physician's practical point of
> view, it is important to know whether they are applicable for clinical
> purposes. Concepts of nonlinear dynamics, fractals, inverse power-law,
> entropy and other terms used in the context with newer analysis
> methods of HR variability refer more to mathematics than to medicine,
> and may be received with some skepticism by clinicians.

In addition, there are methodological limitations in comparing experimental results
to numerical simulations.[40] Nonetheless, evidence for the utility of non-linear
analytical techniques is growing.[41]

Bigger *et al.* computed R–R-interval power spectra in 715 patients with recent
myocardial infarction, 274 healthy persons and 19 patients with heart transplants.[42]
They found that the non-linear spectral scaling properties were a better predictor of
all-cause mortality or arrhythmic death and predicted these outcomes better than
the traditional power spectral bands. In a study of a random sample of 347 elderly
subjects with 10-year follow-up, long-term scaling properties were found to predict
mortality better than traditional HRV. Interestingly, both cardiac and cerebrovas-
cular mortality were predicted. Similarly, in the DIAMOND Study (Danish
Investigations of Arrhythmia and Mortality ON Dofetilide) involving 499 patients
with congestive heart failure and left ventricular ejection fraction $\leq 35\%$, both conventional and fractal HR variability indexes predicted mortality by univariate
analysis.[30] However, after adjusting for age, functional class, medication and left
ventricular ejection fraction in the multivariate proportional-hazards analysis, the
reduced short-term fractal exponent remained the independent predictor of mortality, R–R 1.4 (95% confidence interval (CI) 1.0 to 1.9; $p < 0.05$). In fact, in the
Kaplan–Meier survival curves, higher short-term fractal-scaling exponents had a
significant survival advantage over the lower exponents. This suggests that there
is an intrinsic link between fractal-like dimension of heart rates and survival over

time. Similarly, Tapanainen *et al.* studied heart rate variability and mortality after an acute myocardial infarction in a consecutive series of 806 patients.[43] The patients were divided into two groups based on their left ventricular systolic function (wall motion index), and the predictive power of the short-term scaling exponent (α_1) was analysed in each group. Reduced values of α_1 predicted a significantly increased risk of mortality in both groups (Figure 4.2).

Goldberger *et al.* pointed out that most of the methods utilised to study non-linear behaviour of HRV have been most appropriate for the analysis of mono-fractal signals.[23] Monofractals are homogeneous in the sense that they have the same scaling properties, characterised by only one singularity exponent throughout the entire signal. In contrast, multifractal signals require a larger, and theoretic-ally infinite, number of indices to characterise their scaling properties. His group applied another method to HRV and found that the heart rate time series of healthy humans was multifractal, that this type of complex variability was not simply attributable to physical activity, and that the heart rate time series from patients with severe heart failure show a breakdown of multifractal scaling.[23] Alterations in non-linear measures have been found with other disorders as well, including the metabolic syndrome and diabetes, sleep apnoea, psychiatric disorders such as depression, an oncological disorder – breast cancer – and others.[44–49] In addition to methods based on the R–R interval, other techniques are applicable, such as beat-to-beat Q–T interval variability. Although these and other studies of the predictive power of non-linear methods are compelling, we await intervention trials to demonstrate their clinical usefulness.

Non-linear systems exhibit abrupt transitions. One example of such a transition is a bifurcation in which small changes in a system parameter result in a qualitative change in system behaviour. Variation in the parameter values produces regular oscillations, alternation between two values. Goldberger (and others) have sug-gested that this type of dynamic might underlie a variety of *alternans* patterns in cardiovascular dysfunction, e.g. electrical alternans.[50] Electrical alternans refers to alternate-beat variation in the amplitude and/or morphology of a component of the ECG. True electrical alternans results from repolarisation or a conduction abnor-mality; the electrical alternans observed with pericardial effusion results from motion of the heart. The clinical relevance of this phenomenon is evident from the fact that T-wave or repolarisation alternans appears to be closely associated with the genesis of ventricular arrythmias.[51,52] Although this alternans may be visible to the naked eye on an ECG (Figure 4.3), physiologically important re-polarisation alternans can be too subtle to be detected visually.[51–53] Techniques have been developed to detect microvolt beat-to-beat oscillation of the surface ECG. Rosenbaum *et al.* prospectively studied a group of 83 patients referred for diagnostic electrophysiological testing and found that levels of alternans pre-dicted vulnerability to arrhythmias as defined by the outcomes of both electro-physiological testing and arrhythmia-free survival.[53] In fact, in this study, the presence of such microvolt T-wave alternans detected non-invasively was as strong a predictor of arrhythmia-free survival as invasive electrophysiological testing (Figure 4.4).

Non-linear analytical techniques have been applied not only to 'regular' sinus rhythm, but also to arrhythmias.[54–61] First, non-linear techniques may facilitate the detection and classification of arrhythmias.[62] Second, reduced ventricular re-sponse irregularity is associated with increased mortality in patients with chronic

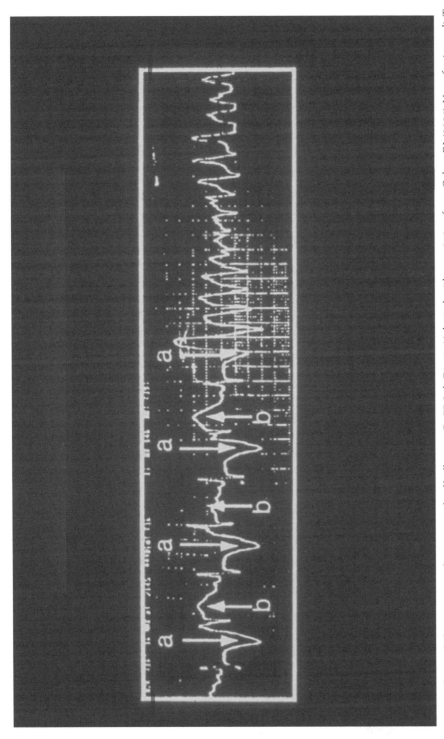

Figure 4.3 Electrical alternans preceding ventricular fibrillation. © *EP Lab Digest*. (Adapted with permission from Cohen RJ (2001) Use of microvolt T-wave alternans testing in clinical practice to reduce sudden cardiac arrest and death. *EP Lab Digest*. **1**: 6–9. www.cambridgeheart.com/camh/ppt/clinical.htm (accessed 16 June 2003).)

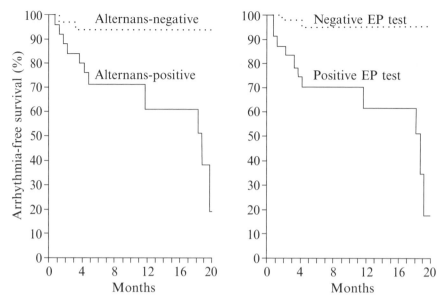

Figure 4.4   T-wave alternans and results of electrophysiologic (EP) testing in relation to arrhythmia-free survival among 66 patients. (a) Arrhythmia-free survival according to Kaplan–Meier life-table analysis is compared with T-wave alternans (alternans ratio > 3.0) and without it (ratio ≤ 3.0). Note that the presence of T-wave alternans is a strong predictor of reduced arrhythmia-free survival. (b) Arrhythmia-free survival among patients with positive EP tests is compared with that among patients in whom ventricular arrhythmias were not induced on EP testing (negative EP test). The predictive value of EP testing and T-wave alternans is essentially the same in these plots. © Mass Med Soc. (Adapted with permission from Rosenbaum DS, Jackson LE, Smith JM, Garan H, Ruskin JN, Cohen RJ (1994) Electrical alternans and vulnerability to ventricular arrhythmias. *N Engl J Med.* **330**: 235–41.)

atrial fibrillation.[63] There is also evidence, albeit mixed, that fibrillation is chaotic.[64] For example, Garfinkel *et al.* examined local extracellular electrograms in three types of haemodynamically stable fibrillation: human atrial fibrillation, canine ventricular fibrillation with maintained coronary blood flow, and ventricular fibrillation in ventricular muscle sheets.[65] They found evidence of an attractor, indicating a chaotic process.[65] The degeneration of tachycardia to fibrillation can be simulated in computer models and a quasiperiodic transition to chaos appears to be a route for this transition.[64] One of the implications is a potential role for non-linear-dynamical arrhythmia control techniques.[56]

For chaotic systems, where behaviour is aperiodic and long-term prediction is impossible, even though the dynamics are entirely deterministic, such determinism can actually be exploited to control the dynamics of a chaotic system. Non-linear dynamical arrhythmia control techniques have been applied successfully in a wide range of physical systems. What is remarkable is that such techniques are model-independent, i.e. they require no a priori knowledge of the underlying equations of a system and are therefore appropriate for systems that are essentially 'black boxes.' These techniques have also been applied in cardiology. While studies in the control of fibrillation in intact hearts has been very limited, there are other arrythmias that lend themselves to this approach, e.g. re-entrant arrhythmias.[66,67]

Control of such dynamics has been demonstrated in computational studies of mathematical arrhythmia models, in vitro rabbit heart experiments and in humans. Christini *et al.* found that in 52 out of 54 control attempts in five patients, an adaptive on-the-fly (i.e. requiring no learning stage) non-linear dynamical control technique could alter cardiac dynamics by simultaneously estimating and stabilising an unstable target rhythm.[60] Control efficacy was not related to antiarrhythmic medications, the presence of dual AV-nodal pathways, or autonomic influences (i.e. control was effective both with and without pharmacological autonomic blockade). Although the findings of this study suggested the feasibility of non-linear dynamical control of cardiac arrhythmias in general, the applicability of this particular control algorithm to arrhythmias other than induced AV-nodal alternans is unclear.

Surprising implications

Just as chaotic systems can produce surprising behaviour, some of the implications of the studies of cardiac rhythms are surprising and counterintuitive. As pointed out by Goldberger and others, conventional physiologic principles dictate that healthy systems are self-regulated to reduce variability and restore constancy – homeostasis.[68] Yet, contrary to the predictions of homeostasis, under healthy conditions, many physiological signals, such as the normal human heartbeat, fluctuate in a complex manner, even under resting conditions. He then suggested that if scale-invariance were a central organising principle of physiological structure and function, we could make a general, but potentially useful prediction about what might happen when these systems are severely perturbed. If a functional system were self-organised in such a way that it does not have a characteristic scale of length or time, a reasonable anticipation would be a breakdown of scale-free structure or dynamics with pathology. Such a breakdown could manifest as either periodic behaviour (one dominant scale) or uncorrelated randomness – complete unpredictability (Figure 4.5). In fact, there are a variety of illnesses that are associated with markedly periodic (regular) behaviour even though the disease states themselves are commonly termed 'dis-orders'.[68] From the most general perspective, the practice of bedside diagnosis itself would be impossible without the loss of complexity and the emergence of pathologic periodicities. To a large extent, it is these periodicities and highly structured patterns – the breakdown of multiscale fractal complexity under pathologic conditions – that allow clinicians to identify and classify many pathologic features of their patients. Familiar examples include periodic tremors in neurologic conditions, AV Wenckebach patterns, the 'sine-wave' ECG pattern in hyperkalaemia, manic-depressive alterations and cyclic breathing patterns in heart failure. A hypothesis was suggested that health is associated with complexity, while disease is associated with complexity loss. Lipsitz suggested that the complex dynamics that represent interacting regulatory processes operating over multiple timescales in good health prime the organism for an adaptive response, making it ready and able to react to sudden physiologic stresses.[69] When the organism is perturbed or deviates from a given set of boundary conditions, most physiological systems evoke closed-loop responses that operate over relatively short periods of time to restore the organism to equilibrium. This transiently alters the dynamics to a less complex, dominant response mode,

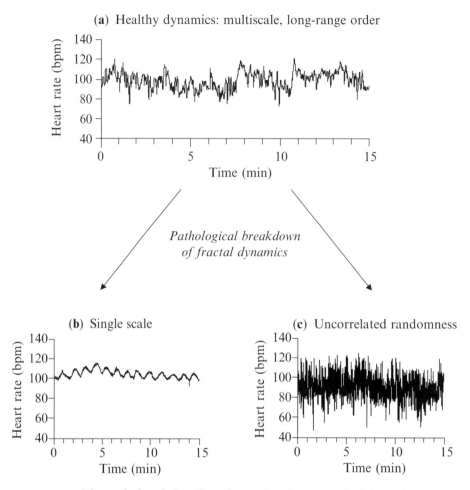

Figure 4.5 Breakdown of a fractal physiological control mechanism can lead ultimately to either a periodic output dominated by a single scale or to uncorrelated randomness. The heart rate series are from: (a) healthy subject; (b) a subject with heart failure; and (c) a subject with atrial fibrillation. © *Lancet*. (Adapted with permission from Goldberger AL (1996) Non-linear dynamics for clinicians: chaos theory, fractals, and complexity at the bedside. *Lancet*. **347**: 1312–14).

which is denoted 'reactive tuning'. Ageing and disease are associated with a loss of complexity in resting dynamics and maladaptive responses to perturbations. These alterations in the dynamics of physiologic systems lead to functional decline and frailty. Whether non-linear mathematical techniques that quantify physiological dynamics may predict the onset of frailty, and interventions aimed toward restoring healthy dynamics could prevent functional decline, remains speculative, and the question will probably not be answered in the near future. However, practical applications of non-linear dynamics are likely within the next few years. The first bedside implementations will be in physiological monitoring. It is important to remember that such monitoring involves at least three agents – patient, staff and monitor. The interactions among them illustrate the second major type of complexity – aggregate complexity.

Aggregate complexity

Aggregate complexity deals with how individual elements work in concert to create systems with complex behaviour. The term *'complex adaptive system'* has been applied in this context. Plsek defines a complex adaptive system as 'a collection of individual agents that have the freedom to act in ways that are not always predictable and whose actions are interconnected such that one agent's actions changes the context for other agents'.[70] Among the attributes of a complex adaptive system are: embeddedness, distributed control, connectivity, co-evolution, non-linearity, dependence on initial conditions and emergent behaviour. Systems are nested in larger systems, many systems contain or include still smaller systems, and sometimes the boundaries of systems overlap. Even in a seemingly hierarchical structure of a single system, there may be no single centralised control mechanism that governs every aspect of system behaviour. The inter-relationships among the adaptive elements of the system produce coherence, but not in a totally predictable fashion, i.e. the whole is greater than the sum of its parts. These inter-relationships mean that an action by one element affects other elements and in turn affects other elements. The effects are not necessarily linear; small changes can have large effects on overall system behaviour, while large changes can have little overall effect. This non-linearity is also associated with sensitivity to initial conditions. Because of the inter-relationships, elements change over time – they co-evolve – and the system patterns of behaviour also change over time. However, these systems are fundamentally unpredictable in their behaviour. Yet, there is the potential for emergent behaviour in complex and unpredictable phenomena – self organization.

The coronary care unit (CCU) is a paradigm of a critical care unit. Characteristics of such units include high levels of staffing and monitoring. They are designed for patients who may be severely ill and at risk of unexpected or at least unpredictable events. Continuous ECG is the most common monitoring procedure and the CCU is a paradigmatic example of a complex adaptive system that has evolved over time. CCUs were established to provide beds with a high level of nursing intensity to which patients with acute coronary syndromes, especially acute myocardial infarction, were admitted. In such units, ECG monitoring and high staff intensity allowed for prompt recognition and treatment of life-threatening arrhythmias. Developments in interventional techniques have resulted in utilisation of such units for early administration of thrombolytic agents, or for urgent coronary angiography and primary angioplasty or stent procedures to salvage myocardial tissue. The rapid evolution of the management of acute coronary syndromes has led to the development of a broader concept of coronary care unit – the integration of acute monitored beds, telemetry-monitored beds and occasionally other beds as well. The CCU is also a small subsystem within the hospital. It is evident that management of patients with acute coronary syndrome involves interactions among multiple disciplines and services. CCUs may be combined with more general intensive care units providing another set of interactions. Moreover, each person in a CCU is a subsystem of that unit and the person, in turn, consists of his/her own subsystems.

In the CCU, the status of the patient is assessed continuously with a variety of monitors, including staff members who observe the patient, the ECG, pulse oximetry and potentially many others. Thus, from a simplistic viewpoint, there are three types of actors – patients, staff and monitoring devices.[71] These three actors interact and adapt to changing contexts. In view of the role of deterministic complexity in evaluation of cardiac rhythms, consider some of the interactions involved in monitoring those rhythms. Although one of the factors driving increasing utilisation of monitoring devices has been to need to relieve the clinical staff from routine tasks, one of the consequences has been a huge increase in the amount of data collected, putting additional cognitive burdens on those same clinical staff. In fact, the modern intensive care unit has been described as a room filled with high-technology patient-monitoring devices whose job it is to report every physiological signal that can possibly be measured.[72] These devices have various means to alert the staff about a problematic situation. Not surprisingly in a room also filled with very ill patients, alarm soundings are frequent. However, many of them are false alarms. In a study of a 10-week period in a paediatric intensive care unit, 86% of the alarms were false alarms.[73] (While intelligent monitoring systems or specialised algorithms utilising non-linear approaches have been proposed to reduce the number of false alarms, the computer/human interface will continue to present challenges.)

Yet, staff must still make decisions. As pointed out by Plsek, in complex adaptive systems, the parts 'have the freedom and ability to respond to stimuli in many different and fundamentally unpredictable ways. For this reason, emergent, surprising, creative behavior is a real possibility. Such behavior can be for better or for worse; that is, it can manifest itself as either innovation or error'.[70] Sometimes, the decisions are quite non-learning, e.g. turning the alarm off and leaving it off! This may reflect that cognitive stress to which the overall intensity of activities contributes, i.e. monitoring occurs in a context. For example, Donchin *et al.* studied a six-bed medical-surgical intensive care unit staffed by a director, a senior attending physician, rotating residents from three different departments and nurses, among others.[74] Twenty-four-hour continuous bedside observations were conducted on a randomly selected group of 46 patients. A total of 8178 activities were observed (an average of 178 per patient per 24 hours). They noted that most of the activities (84%) were performed by a single nurse, while 4.7% of the activities were performed by a single physician, 2.2% by two or more physicians, 2.7% by two nurses, 3% by nurses and physicians, and 3% by others, e.g. technicians and family members. Of note, 33% of the physician activities were classified as reactive rather than planned or initiated. Errors accounted for 0.95% of the activities. The planned activities also reflect interactions among the various actors. On the brighter side, studies of high-reliability teams have found that team members have the ability to monitor each other's activities as a basis for anticipatory task articulation and for pacing of their own activities.[75]

The relevance of deterministic complexity to the CCU can also be illustrated. Pollock found that while traditional analyses of intensive care unit census data failed to reveal patterns, non-linear analyses found characteristics of a chaotic process, including fractal structure.[76] Moreover, the non-linear behaviour of bed occupancy in the CCU (which reflects not only admission rates and activities in the unit and what the patients need, but also the availability of beds in another unit – catherisation lab, surgery, etc.) can result in gridlock. Smooth operation of the CCU can rapidly degenerate into severe congestion as the limit of capacity has been achieved. This is basic to queuing theory. Turner calls this 'Murphy's Curve', because it is at the heart of many of the reasons why systems go wrong.[77]

Summary

The field of complexity studies is broad and heterogeneous. However, several aspects apply to cardiac pathophysiology and to cardiological care delivery. Research along complexity lines has yielded surprising insights into the behaviour of all levels from the individual cell to the cardiac care unit. Moreover, we can anticipate that additional research will necessitate rethinking of some of our basic assumptions.[68,78] It is up to the clinician to be familiar with this field and translate some of the findings into practice.

Acknowledgements

Grateful acknowledgement is given to David S Rosenbaum MD, Director, Heart and Vascular Research Center, MetroHealth Campus, and Jose Ortiz MD, Director, Cardiac Intensive Care Unit, Louis Stokes Cleveland Department of Veterans Affairs Medical Center, Case Western Reserve University School of Medicine, Cleveland, OH, for their helpful comments on the manuscript.

References

1   Rambihar V (1993) Jurassic heart: from the heart to the edge of chaos. *Can Journal of Cardiology.* **9**(9): 787–8.

2   Sataloff RT, Hawkshaw M (2001) *Chaos in Medicine Source Readings.* Singular Publishing Group, San Diego, CA.

3   Stewart I (2002) *Does God Play Dice: the new mathematics of chaos* (2e). Blackwell Publishing, Oxford.

4   The Chaos Hypertextbook – mathematics in the age of the computer. http://hypertextbook.com/chaos/ (accessed 11 June 2003).

5   PhysioNet (2003) www.physionet.org/tutorials/ (accessed 16 June 2003).

6   Denton T, Diamond G, Helfant R *et al.* (1990) Fascinating rhythm: a primer on chaos theory and its application to cardiology. *American Heart Journal.* **120**(6): 1419–40.

7   Wagner C, Persson P (1998) Chaos in the cardiovascular system: an update. *Cardiovascular Research.* **40**(2): 257–64.

8   Liebovitch LS (1998) *Fractals and Chaos Simplified for the Life Sciences.* Oxford University Press, New York.

9   Markovsky B (1998) Social networks and complexity theory. http://cishawaii. org/cis703/files/complexity/markovsky.pdf (accessed 11 June 2003).

10   Phelan SE (2003) What is complexity science really? *Emergence.* **3**(1): 120–36.

11   Manson S (2001) Simplifying complexity: a review of complexity theory. *Geoform.* **32**(3): 405–14.

12   Glenny R, Robertson T, Yamashiro S *et al.* (1991) Applications of fractal analysis to physiology. *Journal of Applied Physiology.* **70**(6): 2351–67.

13   Goldberger AL (1996) Non-linear dynamics for clinicians: chaos theory, fractals, and complexity at the bedside. *Lancet.* **347**(9011): 1312–14.

14   Goldberger A (1992) Fractal mechanisms in the electrophysiology of the heart. *IEEE Engineering in Medicine and Biology.* **3**(2): 47–52.

15 Glenny R, Bernard SL, Robertson HT (2000) Pulmonary blood flow remains fractal down to the level of gas exchange. *Journal of Applied Physiology.* **89**(2): 742–8.

16 Peskin CS, McQueen DM (1994) Mechanical equilibrium determines the fractal fiber architecture of aortic heart value leaflets. *American Journal of Physiology.* **266**(1 Pt 2): H319–H328.

17 Frame M, Mandelbrot B. Fractals in physiology. http://classes.yale.edu/99–00/math190a/Physiology.html (accessed 16 June 2003).

18 Sapoval B, Gobron T, Margolina A (1991) Vibrations of fractal drums. *Physical Review Letters.* **67**(21): 2974–77.

19 Boxt L, Katz J, Czegledy *et al.* (1994) Fractal analysis of pulmonary arteries: the fractal dimension is lower in pulmonary hypertension. *Journal of Thoracic Imaging.* **9**(1): 8–13.

20 Nelson TR, Manchester DK (1988) Modeling of lung cancer morphogenesis using fractal geometries. *IEEE Trans Med Imaging.* **7**(4): 321–7.

21 Bassingthwaighte JB, King RB, Roger SA (1989) Fractal nature of regional myocardial blood flow heterogeneity. *Circ Res.* **65**(3): 578–90.

22 Tsonis AA, Tsonis PA (1987) Fractals: new look at biological shape and patterning. *Perspect Biol Medicine.* **30**(3): 355–61.

23 Goldberger A, Amaral L, Hausdorff J *et al.* (2002) Fractal dynamics in physiology: Alterations with disease and aging. *PNAS.* **99**(suppl. 1): 2466–72.

24 Task Force of the European Society of Cardiology and the North American Society of Pacing and Electrophysiology (1996) Heart rate variability. *European Heart Journal.* **17**(3): 354–81.

25 Cloarec-Blanchard L (1997) Heart rate and blood pressure variability in cardiac diseases: pharmacological implications. *Fundamentals of Clinical Pharmacol.* **11**(1): 19–28.

26 Colhoun H, Francis D, Rubens M *et al.* (2001) The association of heart-rate variability with cardiovascular risk factors and coronary artery calcification: a study in type 1 diabetic patients and the general population. *Diabetes Care.* **24**(12): 1108–14.

27 Gerritsen J, Dekker JM, TenVoorde BJ *et al.* (2001) Impaired autonomic function is associated with increased mortality, especially in subjects with diabetes, hypertension, or history of cardiovascular disease: the Hoorne Study. *Diabetes Care.* **24**(10): 1793–8.

28 Wolf M, Varigos G, Hund D *et al.* (1978) Sinus arrythmia in acute myocardial infarction: two year follow-up. *Medical Journal of Australia.* **2**: 52–3.

29 Mäkikallio T, Tapanainen J, Tulppo M *et al.* (2002) Clinical applicability of heart rate variability by methods based on nonlinear dynamics. *Cardiac Electrophysiology Review.* **6**(3): 250–5.

30 Mäkikallio T, Huikuri H, Hintze U *et al.* (2001) Fractal analysis and time- and frequency-domain measures of heart rate variability as predictors of mortality in patients with heart failure. *American Journal of Cardiology.* **87**(1): 178–82.

31 Tsuji H, Larson MG, Venditti FJ *et al.* (1996) Impact of reduced heart rate variability on risk for cardiac events. The Framingham Heart Study. *Circulation.* **94**(11): 2850–55.

32   Ewing DJ, Campbell IW, Clarke BF (1980) The natural history of diabetic autonomic neuropathy. *Q J Med.* **49**(193): 95–108.

33   Ewing DJ, Borsey DQ, Bellavere F *et al.* (1981) Cardiac autonomic neuropathy in diabetes: comparison of measures of R-R interval variation. *Diabetologia.* **21**(1): 18–24.

34   Lombardi F (2002) Clinical implications of present physiological understanding of HRV components. *Cardiac Electrophysiology Review.* **6**(3): 245–9.

35   Pikkujäsä S, Mäkikallio T, Sourander L *et al.* (1999) Cardiac interbeat interval dynamics from childhood to senescence. *Circulation.* **100**(4): 393–9.

36   Gomes M, Souza A, Guimarães H *et al.* (2000) Investigation of determinism in heart rate variability. *Chaos.* **10**(2): 398–410.

37   Mansier P, Clairambault J, Charlotte N *et al.* (1996) Linear and non-linear analysis of heart rate variability: a mini-review. *Cardiovascular Research.* **31**(3): 371–9.

38   Schumann A, Wessel N, Schirdewan A *et al.* (2002) Potential of feature selection methods in heart rate variability analysis for the classification of different cardiovascular diseases. *Statist Med.* **21**(15): 2225–42.

39   Pincus S (1991) Approximate entropy in cardiology. *Proc Natl Acad Sci USA.* **88**(5): 2297–301.

40   Roth B (2002) Artifacts, assumptions, and ambiguity: pitfalls in comparing experimental results to numerical simulations when studying electrical stimulation of the heart. *American Institute of Physics.* **12**(3): 973–81.

41   Hedman A, Hartikainen J (1999) Has non-linear analysis of heart rate variability any practical value? *Cardiac Electrophysiology Review.* **3**(4): 286–9.

42   Bigger J, Steinman R, Rolnitzky L *et al.* (1996) Power law behavior or RR-interval variability in healthy middle-aged persons, patients with recent acute myocardial infarction, and patients with heart transplants. *Circulation.* **93**(12): 2142–51.

43   Tapanainen J, Thomsen P, Køber L *et al.* (2002) Fractal analysis of heart rate variability and mortality after an acute myocardial infarction. *American Journal of Cardiology.* **90**(4): 347–52.

44   Bettermann H, Kröz M, Girke M *et al.* (2001) Heart rate dynamics and cardiorespiratory coordination in diabetic and breast cancer patients. *Clinical Physiology.* **21**(4): 411–20.

45   Buchman T, Stein P, Goldstein B (2002) Heart rate variability in critical illness and critical care. *Curr Opin Crit Care.* **8**(4): 311–15.

46   Rao R, Yeragani V (2001) Decreased chaos and increased nonlinearity of heart rate time series in patients with panic disorder. *Autonomic Neuroscience: Basic and Clinical.* **88**(1–2): 99–108.

47   Salo T, Kantola I, Voipio-Pulkki L *et al.* (1999) The effect of four different antihypertensive medications on cardiovascular regulation in hypertensive sleep apneic patients – assessment by spectral analysis of heart rate and blood pressure variability. *Fundamentals of Clinical Pharmacol.* **55**(3): 191–8.

48   Trzebski A, Smietanowski M (2001) Non-linear dynamics of cardiovascular system in humans exposed to repetitive apneas modeling obstructive sleep apnea: aggregated time series data analysis. *Autonomic Neuroscience: Basic and Clinical.* **90**(1–2): 106–15.

49 Yeragani V, Radha K, Smitha M *et al.* (2002) Diminished chaos of heart rate time series in patients with major depression. *Biological Psychiatry.* **51**(9): 733–44.

50 Goldberger A (1999) *Nonlinear Dynamics, Fractals, and Chaos Theory: implications for neuroautonomic heart rate control in health and disease.* The Autonomic Nervous System. World Health Organization, Geneva.

51 Pastore J, Girouard S, Laurita K *et al.* (1999) Mechanism linking T-wave alternans to the genesis of cardiac fibrillation. *Circulation.* **99**(10): 1385–94.

52 Walker M, Rosenbaum D (2003) Repolarization alternans: implications for the mechanism and prevention of sudden cardiac death. *Cardiovascular Research.* **57**(3): 599–614.

53 Rosenbaum D, Jackson L, Smith J *et al.* (1994) Electrical alternans and vulnerability to ventricular arrhythmias. *New England Journal of Medicine.* **330**(4): 235–41.

54 Amann A, Achleitner U, Antretter H *et al.* (2001) Analyzing ventricular fibrillation ECG-signals and predicting defibrillation success during cardiopulmonary resuscitation employing N(a)-histograms. *Resuscitation.* **50**(1 July): 77–85.

55 Biktashev V, Holden A (2001) Characterization of patterned irregularity in locally interacting, spatially extended systems: ventricular fibrillation. *Chaos.* **11**(3): 653–64.

56 Christini D, Glass L (2002) Mapping and control of complex cardiac arrhythmias. *Chaos.* **12**(3): 732–9.

57 Hastings H, Evans S, Quan W *et al.* (1996) Nonlinear dynamics in ventricular fibrillation. *Proc Natl Acad Sci USA.* **93**(19): 10 495–9.

58 Stein P (2003) Heart rate turbulence: explorations of an emerging risk factor. *Journal of Cardiovasc Electrophysiol.* **14**(5): 453–54.

59 Stein P, Schmieg R, El-Fouly A *et al.* (2001) Association between heart rate variability recorded on postoperative day 1 and length of stay in abdominal aortic surgery patients. *Crit Care Medicine.* **29**(9): 1738–43.

60 Christini D, Stein K, Markowitz S *et al.* (1995) Nonlinear-dynamical arrhythmia control in humans. *Proc Natl Acad Sci USA.* **98**(10): 5827–32.

61 Garfinkel A, Weiss J, Ditto W *et al.* (1995) Chaos control of cardiac arrhythmias. *Trends in Cardiovascular Medicine.* **5**(2): 76–80.

62 Owis M, Abou-Zied A, Youssef A *et al.* (2002) Study of features based on nonlinear dynamical modeling in ECG arrhythmia detection and classification. *IEEE Trans Biomed Eng.* **49**(7): 733–6.

63 Yamada A, Hayano J, Sakata S *et al.* (2000) Reduced ventricular response irregularity is associated with increased mortality in patients with chronic atrial fibrillation. *Circulation.* **102**(3): 300–6.

64 Weiss J, Garfinkel A, Karagueuzian H *et al.* (1999) Chaos and the transition to ventricular fibrillation. *Circulation.* **99**(64): 2819–26.

65 Garfinkel A, Chen P, Walter D *et al.* (1997) Quasiperiodicity and chaos in cardiac fibrillation. *Journal of Clinical Investigation.* **99**(2): 305–14.

66 Hastings H, Fenton F, Evans S *et al.* (2000) Alternans and the onset of ventricular fibrillation. *Physical Review E.* **62**(3): 4043–8.

67 Nearing B, Verrier R (2002) Progressive increases in complexity of T-wave oscillations herald ischemia-induced ventricular fibrillation. *Circulation.* **91**(8): 727–32.

68 Goldberger AL (1997) Fractal variability versus pathologic periodicity: complexity loss and stereotype in disease. *Perspect Biol Medicine.* **40**(4): 543–61.

69 Lipsitz L (2002) Dynamics of stability: the physiologic basis of functional health and frailty. *Journals of Gerontology.* **57A**(3): B115–B125.

70 Plsek P (2001) Redesigning health care with insights from the science of complex adaptive systems. In: P Plsek. *Crossing the Quality Chasm: A New Health System for the 21st Century.* The National Academy of Sciences, Washington, DC, pp. 309–17.

71 Walsh T, Beatty P (2002) Human factors error and patient monitoring. *Physiological Measurement.* **23**(3): R111–R132.

72 Tsien C (1997) Reducing false alarms in the intensive care unit: systematic comparison of four algorithms. http://medicine.ucsd.edu/f97/D004115.htm (accessed 11 June 2003).

73 Tsien C, Fackler J (1997) Poor prognosis for existing monitors in the intensive care unit. *Crit Care Medicine.* **25**(4): 614–19.

74 Donchin A, Gopher D, Olin M *et al.* (1995) A look into the nature and causes of human errors in the intensive care unit. *Crit Care Medicine.* **23**: 294–300.

75 Xiao Y (2001) Practices of high reliability terms: observations in trauma resuscitation. *Proceedings of the Human Factors and Ergonomics Society*, Baltimore, MD, pp. 395–9.

76 Pollock JE (2003) Using nonlinear analysis to describe and forecast the patient census of an intensive care unit. http://southerct.edu/chaos-nursing/abstracts.htm (accessed 11 June 2003).

77 Turner S, Robinson S, Seeley D (2003) Avoiding crisis culture: visualizing the deep structure of health care capacity. http://itch.uvic.ca/itch2000/TURNER/TURNER.HTM (accessed 11 June 2003).

78 Glass L (2001) Synchronization and rhythmic processes in physiology. *Nature.* **410**: 277–84.

CHAPTER 5

Complexity and diabetes

Tim Holt

Everyday life with diabetes involves a complex interaction between numerous influences determining the way the person feels and the success with which the markers of good health are kept within acceptable limits. These not only include blood glucose levels, but also lipids, weight, blood pressure, and indices of social health and wellbeing, which for many are at least equally important. Blood glucose control is therefore just one issue embedded in a wider context of different and sometimes competing priorities in the individual.

Patients vary markedly in the priority they give to tight glycaemic control, and in their attitude towards self-monitoring. Once the overall daily insulin dose and its distribution through the day are established, many patients choose not to 'tamper' with the system but accept that on days when (perhaps) exercise levels are higher, they will require more carbohydrate (CHO) or less insulin, and make adjustments accordingly, relying not on monitoring but on symptoms to warn them if their decisions have displaced the system too far. This approach, which aims to simply replace the missing insulin, might be the best one for some individuals, particularly if the average blood glucose level, based on HbA1c estimation, is satisfactory and hypoglycaemia awareness is intact.

But for patients whose lifestyle needs to be more flexible (in whom variation in exercise or CHO intake is wider or more frequent), for those with reduced awareness of hypo- or hyperglycaemic symptoms, or in those who have decided that merely 'satisfactory' Hba1c levels are not acceptable (an increasing proportion of patients), more needs to be done to replace the other missing component in the system – the regulation mechanism that maintains euglycaemia in the physiological state. This chapter will explore this area from the perspective of complexity.

Understanding blood glucose dynamics

The dynamics of blood glucose variation are difficult to investigate, for a number of reasons. Many of the determinants (particularly exercise levels) are difficult to quantify. Serial measurements of blood glucose need to be taken frequently to make any sense of the dynamics, which in real-life situations may differ from those in more controlled conditions. Blood glucose behaviour may be non-stationary – the statistical properties may vary over time within an individual – and patients may differ in a number of ways that make research conclusions difficult to generalise.

Limitations of linear models

A standard measure of glycaemic control is the glycosylated haemoglobin (HbA1c) level, an easily measurable index that reflects *average* blood glucose levels over a period of about three months. HbA1c levels have transformed the monitoring of glycaemic control, but give no information at all about dynamical behaviour. Two patients may have similar HbA1c levels, one with a relatively static profile, the other with widely fluctuating levels around the same mean value. Clinicians or patients may examine blood glucose profiles retrospectively to try to understand the dynamics, but it is difficult to make much sense of them when so much information on the core blood glucose determinants (such as carbohydrate intake and exercise levels) is usually missing.[1] These dynamical properties are important, first because highly variable or rapidly changing levels around a satisfactory mean implies that control may in fact be inadequate (the patient may be spending significant periods in the hypoglycaemic range), and conversely, that an apparently disorderly profile might in fact reflect orderly underlying processes.

Like the HbA1c, blood glucose levels themselves are objective and accurately measurable. How useful are such levels on their own in understanding the dynamics and predicting outcomes? The answer seems to depend on the model used. The autocorrelation function is a linear measure of correlation between successive values. Through studying published data from frequently recorded blood glucose measurements in a variety of settings (including non-diabetics as well as type 1 and type 2 patients) Bremer and Gough[2] found that measurements correlate within a time frame of no more than about 10 minutes. This sets a limit on the usefulness of blood glucose levels alone as a key to understanding the dynamics using linear models, except for the recognition of impending hypoglycaemia. It also means there is insufficient published data involving such frequent measurements. In soliciting the collection of more data, the authors conclude:

> The success of linear models in predicting glycemic dynamics indicates that such models may be used in conjunction with frequent blood glucose measurements to provide an earlier warning of impending hypoglycemia than would be attainable by measurement alone. However, a simple linear model created from a single day of blood glucose measurements is not expected to be applicable for predicting blood glucose dynamics without being updated. Since the biological processes responsible are nonlinear and nonstationary under many conditions, models that are more complex are expected to improve the predictor performance and extend the prediction horizon. However, these models will require more data collected over long periods of time from more individuals than is currently available in the literature.

Can complexity assist in the development of such models? There are a number of possible ways that it might, namely:

- the inclusion of more variables
- recognising *interactions* between these variables
- utilising the concept of a *phase space* of blood glucose determinants
- assessing the system's behaviour using non-linear time series analysis.

A phase space model for blood glucose variation

In Chapter 1 we saw how Lorenz's simplified model of a weather system produced chaotic behaviour – behaviour that is apparently random when one variable is assessed alone, but quite orderly when all the variables are plotted in phase space. So let's imagine the blood glucose level and its 'core' determinants (CHO intake, insulin levels, exercise levels and insulin sensitivity) as axes in a phase space. This gives us five dimensions – too many for a page in this book, so let us reduce it down to just three variables by imagining that exercise level is zero or at a constant low background level and that insulin sensitivity is stable (Figures 5.1 and 5.2). These diagrams give us an idea of how we might apply the phase space concept to blood glucose behaviour but, as discussed below, a complete description of the system would need to also include their rates of change (as these also determine the way the system evolves), adding even more axes.

Figure 5.1 shows the current state of the system, a single point plotted using the values of the coordinate variables at a given moment in time. In Figure 5.2, this point becomes a trajectory, as the values for each variable change. This gives us an idea of 'where the system is' at any one time (the current position) and its evolution over time. We could calculate the average value of each variable, and their ranges of values, but the phase space gives us much more information than that. It gives us an idea of the combinations of values that tend to occur together and the geometrical properties of the trajectory over time – the properties of the systems *attractor*. These are the key to understanding the system's dynamics. The rest of this chapter explores where this model might take us both in helping patients to improve control and in measuring their success.

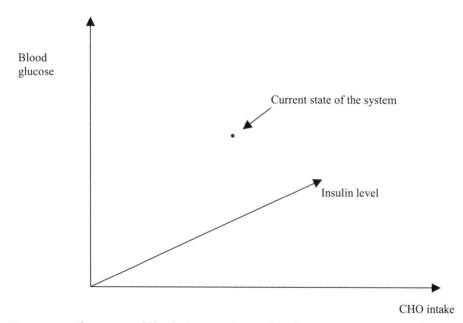

Figure 5.1   Phase space of blood glucose and two of its determinants.

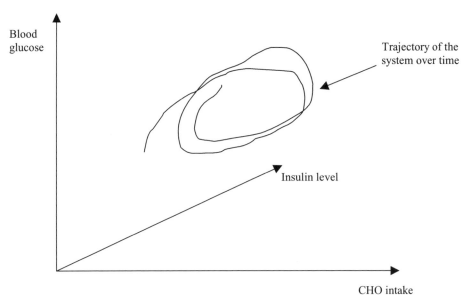

Figure 5.2 Trajectory of the system moving through three dimensions over time.

Statistical versus deterministic approaches

Patients aiming to control their blood glucose levels tightly use information about initial conditions (i.e. the values of the current blood glucose and its determinants) to predict what is likely to happen next. Advice, or decisions about 'what to expect next' or 'what to do next', are usually based on statistical probabilities, recognising the inevitable chance element that results from unknown or unquantified variables in the system. According to this model, the uncertainty in outcomes could be reduced to arbitrarily low levels by examining enough examples of similar scenarios (i.e. by taking a large enough sample from a randomly distributed population of similar states). In other words, we use a statistical approach to base our expectations and decisions on a perceived *average trajectory*, perhaps gleaned through the patient's long personal experience of his/her own blood glucose behaviour, perhaps actually calculated through examining past data, and the more of it available the lower the uncertainty and the better will be the predictions. This approach is perfectly accessible to an external agent such as a clinician, who can perhaps see that of the last eight examples in the past month where the blood glucose level was around 5 mmol/l before tea, the blood glucose at bedtime was consistently higher than is acceptable. Conclusion: insufficient short-acting insulin covering the evening meal.

Berger *et al.* have utilised this principle to develop a computer-based tool for optimising the insulin regimen, called CADMO.[3] By calculating average blood glucose levels at specified times of day retrospectively over a period of weeks, and using a physiological model of insulin kinetics, the tool is able to explore a large space of possible combinations of insulin types and doses to select the regimen that is most likely, on an average day, to render the glucose level constant. As a complement to the 'human expert', this tool makes use of the computer's ability to process and analyse large volumes of data.

This might be called the *statistical approach* and it bases expectations on 'average' behaviour. It is the same approach used more generally when a clinician offers evidence-based advice to a patient about treatment options, assuming that although the patient is a unique individual, he or she belongs to a randomly distributed population similar to that from which the evidence has been derived, and will *on average* respond to the treatment in the way predicted.[4]

But the study of chaos lends us another possibility: that while the iteration of a *simple* algorithm might determine the new values for the variables over time, the uniqueness of the starting conditions and the system's sensitivity to initial conditions mean that no amount of studying past behaviour will reduce the uncertainty beyond a short time horizon, as the uncertainty is an inherent property of the system and not the result of unknown or chance factors. This might be called the *deterministic approach*, and is explained further in Figure 5.3 and Box 5.1.

To emphasise this distinction, I quote the philosopher Stephen Kellert from his very balanced account of the impact of chaos theory on modern thinking, *In The Wake of Chaos:*[5]

> ... a system is deterministic if the dynamical system that models it makes no reference to chance. ... Any complex behaviour in the dynamical system must come from its internal mathematical structure, not from the fact that the system is an approximation of a huge number of complicated interacting subsystems. The deterministic approach chaos theory takes to the study of apparently disorderly behaviour is thus in contrast to a statistical approach, which focuses on the evolution of average values at many places in the system, or averages over many systems.

So as well as analysing information from past scenarios, patients might also make predictions by executing a sort of 'algorithm' determining a projected trajectory

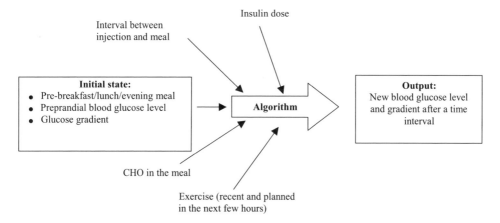

Figure 5.3 An algorithm determining the new blood glucose level and gradient as a function of a number of inputs. Whilst the inputs are few enough to be consciously processed by the patient, they are easily numerous enough that comparable combinations will be rarely found in a historical profile, even if the appropriate information were recorded. Non-linear effects enter due to interactions between the inputs – the exercise level modifies the effect of insulin, which also depends on initial blood glucose levels, but the model is still relatively simple, and complex behaviour may arise because of this non-linearity, not because the number of inputs is large.

Box 5.1 Deterministic chaos in the Lorenz model

Lorenz demonstrated *chaos* in a simplified model of a weather system, producing the beautiful attractor pattern displayed on the cover of this book. The properties of this attractor can only be fully appreciated when the trajectory is seen to develop in real time, so readers may wish to visit:

www.sat.t.u-tokyo.ac.jp/~hideyuki/java/Attract.html

This is an example, to use the title of his paper, of 'deterministic non-periodic flow'.[6] The trajectory never settles to a steady state, but never repeats itself. To create this pattern Lorenz defined his system (in fact an idealised chamber containing air with a temperature gradient applied across it) using three differential equations, three system variables and three model parameters. Each point on the attractor is determined (completely) by feeding the values of the system's variables from the time step before it into these equations. The next step is then determined by reiterating this process using the current values, and so on. The future trajectory is determined indefinitely into the future by the starting position, but because of sensitivity to measurement error in these initial conditions, it cannot be predicted beyond a short time horizon. The only way of finding out the future course is to apply repeated iterations to the equations and watch what happens. In the very short term, outcomes are predictable as a function of the initial conditions. But the medium-term behaviour does not represent an approximation of 'average' outcomes developing from similar starting conditions; examining even a large sample of past examples will not help us in predicting outcomes beyond this time horizon. However, the existence of determinism and the low dimension of the attractor mean that structure is apparent that usefully distinguishes chaos from randomness over short time periods.

---

over a short timescale. The initial state represents the current blood glucose level, its rate of change with respect to time (the glucose gradient) and the time of day; inputs are the CHO in the forthcoming meal, the insulin dose before it, the interval between injection and the meal, and the exercise completed and planned a few hours either side of it; the output is the blood glucose level and gradient at the next time step. The aim is to adjust the modifiable inputs to produce a normal blood glucose level at the next time step. While accepting a chance element, this approach depends on a deterministic relationship between relatively few inputs and the output (Figure 5.3).

If we assumed that the system were perfectly linear: that changes in blood glucose levels resulted from a simple summation of independent influx and efflux effects (CHO intake and insulin doses or exercise, respectively), and particularly if the glucose gradient were not an issue (an assumption made in most models), then a retrospective statistical analysis of past data would be a reasonable approach to guide control and dose adjustment. But if, like a bank account with compound interest, non-linear interactions are introduced, then a system with even a small number of variables may become complex, and future behaviour cannot easily be predicted even if the interactions are perfectly understood.

To what extent is each approach beneficial to individual patients with diabetes? No one could deny the role of chance factors in blood glucose variation, but there is an important issue here about the usefulness of historical blood glucose profiles in aiding decision making, and the best source of guidance for individual patients.

Non-stationary system parameters

One of the problems with either of the above approaches is that complex systems rarely 'stay still' for very long. Variation in the systems' *parameters* makes it difficult to maintain predictability, as these parameters change (like the bank's interest rate might) over longer timescales than the variables. In diabetes, this might equate to a change in insulin sensitivity over time, perhaps due to a change in the patient's weight. These more gradual changes mean than the algorithms that determine the structure of trajectories through phase space will need adjusting over time. This, in practice, will require an awareness of the system's movement over this timescale.

This opens up the concept of 'ageing data'. Liszka-Hackzell[7] studied a blood glucose profile from an insulin-treated patient involving at least twice-daily measurements over two years. His model was trained using this data and was able to make successful predictions over a period of 15 days, but after this period predictability was lost and the model would have required retraining on a weekly basis using recent data in order to track the non-stationary properties. While this study involved only one individual, it raises the question over the validity of advice given in clinics to type 1 patients beyond a two-week timescale.

In practice, patients aiming to keep blood glucose within close limits might apply both strategies, recognising the uniqueness of each situation and its pattern of starting conditions, and at the same time utilising information from past behaviour to predict the future trajectory. Can we join these approaches together, combining both under the same model? The next section describes how this might be achieved.

The snooker cue – a non-linear metaphor for glycaemic control

Lorenz's insights have been applied to his own field of meteorology, in which the system's behaviour, on a scale that affects our daily lives considerably, is predictable only within a short time horizon (at least in the UK). But one of the crucial distinctions between diabetes management and weather prediction is that while meteorologists measure initial conditions (today's temperature, wind speed, air pressure, etc.) to make short-term predictions (tomorrow's weather), action taken as a result of the prediction doesn't significantly affect the outcome. Wearing a raincoat tomorrow on the weather forecaster's advice may affect whether or not we get wet, but it won't affect whether or not it rains. This situation might conceivably change in the future if the weather became controllable, but for the time being there is only one direction of influence.

But patients who self-monitor are not only measuring initial conditions to understand where the system is 'right now', and perhaps where it is liable to go over the next few hours, they are also likely to act on this information in such a way that might alter the outcomes considerably. Indeed, this is why many patients do it. They are not simply taking measurements to show to a clinician a month later. They are hoping to offset impending hypoglycaemia, or decide how much CHO to take before exercise, or perhaps how much insulin they need to cover the next meal. Such patients are, in a sense, locked into a coupled feedback loop through which awareness of blood glucose levels affects behaviour, and vice versa. The effect of this awareness is difficult to include in the development of optimisation tools such as CADMO, or indeed clinician-based advice, but can make all the difference between success and failure in tight control strategies.

As I have argued in previous work[8,9] the traditional metaphor for 'balance' in diabetes control has been the *weighing scales*, a model in which a linear equivalence principle is assumed between carbohydrate intake and insulin doses, or carbohydrate intake and exercise. This model on its own tends to ignore the system's dynamism, and fails to recognise that all three components need to be weighed up simultaneously and that the components may interact with each other. It also has difficulty incorporating the concept of non-stationarity, which as we have seen, may be a significant problem for individuals even though it is a healthy feature of normal physiology. This metaphor may be appropriate for patients who can achieve a flat baseline insulin level, and the advent of long-acting insulin analogues and continuous subcutaneous insulin infusions are making this baseline state a real possibility. This has caused something of a revival in the weighing scales metaphor and an emphasis on accuracy of measurement through the DAFNE (Dose Adjustment For Normal Eating) programme.[10] For those who can achieve an equilibrium condition in which preprandial blood glucose and insulin levels are flat, and who are motivated to accurately calculate CHO intake, this approach may be the best option.

A more dynamic and perhaps realistic metaphor, at least for type 1 patients, is that of the *snooker cue*,[9] balanced on the palm of the hand or the tip of the finger, a model inspired by the mathematician Ian Stewart.[11] This model attempts to account for inevitable movement, rather than ignore it. The cue moves in three dimensions simultaneously; removing one of these dimensions (perhaps by placing the hand on a table surface, removing the up/down dimension) makes control of the cue's position more, not less, difficult. The roughly upright position of the cue can be set by an external assistant, corresponding in glycaemic control to the identification of the broad parameters of the system, such as the overall daily insulin requirement appropriate for the patient's weight and insulin sensitivity, and its approximate distribution through the day. But beyond this, only the cue balancer knows what immediate responses will be required to maintain the upright position. This model not only recognises, but it also *values* dynamism, because even though the balancer is continually attempting to avoid over-correction, movement is, in a sense, part of the control mechanism.

Balance is maintained through a partly intuitive skill, frequent proprioceptive feedback on the current position and an ability to harness the movement where appropriate but minimise it otherwise. While the weighing scales model relies for success on *accuracy of measurement* (of CHO, exercise and insulin doses), the snooker cue relies on *feedback and an awareness of movement*, recognising (as meteorologists do) that even highly accurate measurements of initial conditions will not extend the predictive horizon very much. Examining past examples of similar cue positions (even if the balancer had time to do so) would give little reliable guidance on what to do next. Simple rules applied intuitively are more effective in this situation than an analysis of past behaviour as a guide to immediate action.

Divergence or convergence?

There are a number of assumptions made in developing this argument. One is that trajectories in glycaemic phase space tend to diverge rather than converge. The snooker cue itself diverges for fairly obvious reasons – similar but non-identical starting positions will become less similar over time, as gravity attracts the cue in slightly different directions in either case. But this property might not necessarily apply to patients with diabetes.

In type 1 disease, where survival is dependent on taking insulin injections, the behaviour of the individual is part of the regulation mechanism. Appropriate dosing and timing of insulin, CHO intake and exercise are essential components, liable to be influenced by blood glucose monitoring, blood glucose levels themselves (which if high might reduce the exercise expenditure due to lethargy) and hypo/hyperglycaemia awareness, which might be misinterpreted, causing inappropriate action. Correction of hypoglycaemia with fast-acting CHO may cause hyperglycaemia, followed by an increase in insulin dose higher than is required, repeating the cycle. All these interactions create the possibility of positive feedback effects, in which a disturbance to the system becomes amplified over time due to secondary behavioural mechanisms. Particularly in patients aiming for tight control, there is an *inherent instability* in the system.

Type 2 diabetes controlled by diet or oral hypoglycaemics on the other hand involves more complex pathophysiology[12] and, perhaps largely due to the existence of residual insulin excretion, the system contains a degree of self-correction. Such patients are on the whole likely to have trajectories that *converge*, albeit to a displaced attracting point set towards the hyperglycaemic range. In such patients, a resetting of this baseline position is the major goal; the system is liable to converge back towards it following displacement. Self-monitoring therefore takes a lower priority and is more difficult to justify routinely in type 2 patients.[13]

Avoiding over-correction

Practice at actually balancing a snooker cue on the palm reveals two quite distinct extremes of behaviour, both compatible with maintaining the cue roughly upright. One is smooth, the other is jerky and erratic. *In both cases, the 'average' position is vertically upright.*

The first of these two behaviours represents an appropriate response to the proprioceptive signals indicating the cue's current position and likely immediate trajectory. This trajectory is predictable in the very short term but, other than predicting that the cue will remain roughly upright indefinitely, there is no saying exactly which position it will be in a few seconds later. Each 'state' is determined by the state a short time interval before it, and the cue's movement, while unpredictable over longer timescales, is not random. This pattern is characteristic of low-dimensional chaotic variation.

The other, more erratic behaviour results from an inappropriate over-reaction to these proprioceptive signals, due to inexperience or lack of skill. In this situation, there is no structure, even to the short-term variation, because the potentially low-dimensional variation is being disrupted externally. This corresponds to the maladaptive responses patients may make to frequent self-monitoring, and the resulting variation becomes less distinguishable from random noise. Even though the cue is still moving in three physical dimensions, the dynamics are high-dimensional and therefore closer to random noise. This erratic movement is therefore (perhaps counterintuitively) *less chaotic* in the stricter sense of the term, through its lack of low-dimensional determinism.

These different behaviours of the cue might be studied in the way that engineers have studied similar physical non-linear systems. Could we use the same techniques in patients with diabetes to identify healthy, smooth and adaptive movement through glycaemic phase space, and distinguish it from the more random and structureless pattern?

Reconstructing an attractor using just one system variable

The phase space model lends itself to study using non-linear time series analysis. But we are still faced with the problem of unquantifiable variables. In glycaemic phase space, insulin doses and blood glucose levels may be accurately recorded, CHO intake less so, but exercise levels are notoriously difficult to quantify in real-life situations. And erratic insulin absorption means that insulin doses bear an inconsistent relationship to plasma insulin profiles. How can we get around this problem?

In the early 1980s, Floris Takens and David Ruelle discovered a way of reconstructing an attractor using only one of the system's variables. They suggested that instead of plotting a phase space defined by each variable, we take a time series of just one variable, and plot successive values separated by standard time delays as each axis. They showed that the geometrical properties of the resulting attractor (including the correlation dimension and the Lyapunov exponents) are the same as the attractor defined by plotting all the system's variables. This principle is explained in brief by Ian Stewart,[11] who describes how the Lorenz attractor can be reconstructed in this way (pp. 172–4), and more technically by Schaffer.[14] There is no guarantee that this technique would necessarily work for a blood glucose time series, but the approach provides a possible solution to the problem mentioned early in this chapter — the need for a more complex underlying model to represent blood glucose dynamics that still uses blood glucose levels alone (see Figure 5.4).

This means, at least in theory, that the dimension of the attractor might be measured using only blood glucose levels. A time series of frequent blood glucose measurements might indicate how large the space is in which the blood glucose level is embedded. This could then be measured in a number of different scenarios, including type 1 and type 2 patients at different times, and most importantly, indicate the effect of an awareness of the monitoring results on the dynamics of blood glucose variation. A reduction in the dimension from a high level (indicating effectively random variation) to low-dimensional movement might provide evidence, on dynamical rather than statistical grounds, of the success of self-monitoring in the individual. Conversely, a shift in the opposite

Blood
glucose
level
at time
$(t + T)$

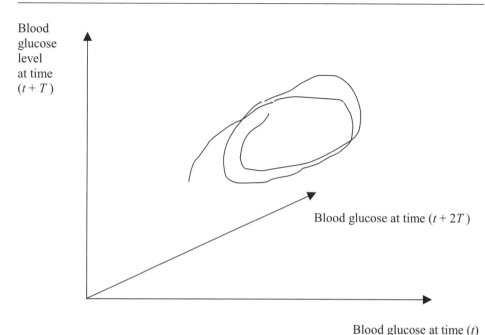

Blood glucose at time $(t + 2T)$

Blood glucose at time (t)

Figure 5.4   Embedding a blood glucose time series to reconstruct an attractor, showing three
dimensions. The axes represent the blood glucose values after successive time intervals T.
The geometrical properties of this attractor are similar to those of the attractor defined by all
the system's determinant variables. In this way, these properties might be measured even though
only the blood glucose levels are accurately known.

direction might be an indication of poor control strategies and a maladaptive
response to monitoring. The Lyapunov exponents, which are a measure of the
tendency of trajectories to diverge from close starting positions, might indicate the
inherent instability of the system in an individual, the impact on this of self-
monitoring, and give an estimate of the predictive time horizon. This approach
revives the concept of 'brittleness' as an inherent property of an individual's
diabetes, and might make it measurable in a more meaningful way than previously
possible. In practice, the use of such techniques in studying physiological time
series is difficult, and the data are often too noisy to detect underlying
deterministic processes,[15] but might still be worth exploring now that frequent
monitoring is relatively easy in everyday circumstances.

Kroll[16] has applied these techniques retrospectively to blood glucose and insulin
level time series, and detected four-dimensional structure with directional flow in
phase space and positive Lyapunov exponents, indicating a component of
deterministic chaos. This gives an impetus to the application of these techniques
more widely in diabetes research using data from a variety of patient types in
different circumstances.

Chaotic control

Patients displaying *sensitivity to initial conditions* will have trajectories that tend
to diverge from close starting points, i.e. minor disturbances to the system tend to

become amplified so that similar but non-identical starting conditions become less similar over time, like the movement of the snooker cue. In correcting this tendency, the cue-balancer intuitively carries out an 'operation' on the system:

- receiving feedback on the current position
- making short-term predictions about the likely future course in all three dimensions (i.e. the immediate trajectory)
- adjusting the position not directly to the 'desired' upright position (as this would cause over-correction), but in a way that recognises that the system is moving.

This operation needs to be done either continuously or at sequential intervals that are comparable with the system's predictive time horizon. While Bremer and Gough[2] found that the linear autocorrelation function is only significant over time periods of about 10 minutes, this timescale might be extended through the inclusion of other system variables. Riva and Bellazzi[17] analysed historical profiles from eight type 1 patients using three different Bayesian techniques and were able to derive a model for predicting blood glucose levels one step ahead (i.e. the time interval between sequential injections on a four-times-a-day regimen). Interestingly, all three techniques selected as the best model the *simplest* one using relatively few inputs.

This type of operation is reminiscent of that used in a classical experiment by Garfinkel *et al.*,[18] in which chaotic contractions in an isolated rabbit myocardium were rendered periodic using a similar principle. The researchers recorded measurements of interbeat intervals and were able to recognise structure in a two-dimensional phase space, whose axes represented the current interval and the following interval (i.e. using the same embedding principle described above). They then identified 'stable manifolds' – directions in phase space that would tend to carry the system towards the desired periodic point (the central point in the diagram where both intervals are equal) – and, by stimulating the myocardium at the appropriate moments, nudged the system recurrently back towards these manifolds rather than directly towards the desired point, to avoid over-correction. The success of the technique was dramatically demonstrated when the mechanism was switched on and off, causing the sudden appearance and disappearance of periodic contractions respectively.

This is a well-known example of 'chaotic control'. Garfinkel's group commented that a problem they encountered was a shift in the stable manifolds over time. This non-stationary effect would need to be accounted for by redefining the manifolds using feedback of recent behaviour. This is reminiscent of the problem encountered by Liszka-Hackzell, who found that his predictions of blood glucose behaviour would require continual retraining using recent results in order to remain valid in the face of ageing data.[7]

Because the very process of responding to proprioceptive signals is a potential source of instability, control of blood glucose using this approach is only likely to succeed if:

- the broad parameters of the system (such as total daily insulin dose) are fairly accurately set (using the statistical approach). Fine control of the snooker cue is only possible when the cue is roughly upright

- adjustments made to the variables are minor
- monitoring is continuous rather than a brief or 'one-off' exercise
- movement is recognised and valued as a source of flexibility and control, but minimised
- consistent non-stationary trends can be distinguished from random variation effects.

The success of this model in improving over the 'don't tamper' approach of setting the system's broad parameters and then resisting the temptation to interfere, depends on the existence of low-dimensional structure in the dynamics, as well as the patient's skill. If the dynamics were high dimensional or frankly random, then the 'don't tamper' approach might be more appropriate. A device attached to the cue to introduce vibrations as a source of noise would effectively scupper any attempts to respond appropriately to this variation, which would simply have to be accepted. But this would depend on the relative amplitude of the noise, and on the balancer's ability to distinguish it from the smoother movement – to separate the low-dimensional structure from the high-dimensional disruption. This distinction would need to be made on *qualitative* rather than quantitative grounds. The exciting prospect is that this area of diabetes research is becoming accessible through the advent of very frequent monitoring technology in real-life situations and the use of non-linear time series analysis.

Summary

The principles of complexity and non-linear dynamics might be applied to diabetes care in a number of ways. Non-linear models of blood glucose variation might allow the dynamism in the system to be recognised and appreciated as a lever for glycaemic control. Non-linear interactions between the determinants of blood glucose might be seen as an intrinsic source of unpredictability, placing a limit on our ability to reduce variation. Sources of order, including low-dimensional determinism might be recognised as useful tools in achieving tight control. And research techniques now established in other fields might assess the adequacy of control and the influence of self-monitoring from a dynamical perspective. Above all, complex non-linear models of type 1 diabetes recognise that an element of control, perhaps an essential element for *tight* control, is only accessible to the individual patient, who witnesses the dynamics from within the system on a continuous basis. Such patients may benefit from statistical approaches both in setting the broad parameters of the system and adjusting them in response to non-stationary effects, but immediate decision making may depend more reliably on simple deterministic rules applied intuitively over short timescales than on analysis of historical profiles that may soon become outdated.

Acknowledgement

I am grateful to Barry Tennison for his useful comments on an earlier draft of this chapter.

References

1 Wilson T, Holt T, Greenhalgh T (2001) Complexity science: complexity and clinical care. *BMJ.* **323**: 685–8.

2 Bremer T, Gough DA (1999) Is blood glucose predictable from previous values? A solicitation for data. *Diabetes.* **48**: 445–51.

3 Berger MP, Gelfand RA, Miller PL (1990) Combining statistical, rule-based, and physiologic model-based methods to assist in the management of diabetes mellitus. *Computers and Biomedical Research.* **23**: 346–57.

4 Sackett DL, Straus SE, Scott Richardson W *et al.* (2000) *Evidence-based Medicine: how to teach and practice EBM* (2e). Churchill Livingstone, London.

5 Kellert SH (1993) *In the Wake of Chaos.* University of Chicago Press, Chicago.

6 Lorenz EN (1963) Deterministic non-periodic flow. *Journal of the Atmospheric Sciences.* **20**: 130–41.

7 Liszka-Hackzell JJ (1999) Prediction of blood glucose levels in diabetic patients using a hybrid AI technique. *Computers and Biomedical Research.* **32**: 132–44.

8 Holt TA (2002) A chaotic model for tight diabetes control. *Diabetic Medicine.* **19**: 274–8.

9 Holt TA (2003) Non-linear dynamics and diabetes control. *The Endocrinologist.* **13**(6): 452–6.

10 DAFNE Study Group (2002) Training in flexible, intensive insulin management to enable dietary freedom in people with type 1 diabetes: dose adjustment for normal eating (DAFNE) randomised controlled trial *BMJ.* **325**: 746.

11 Stewart I (1990) *Does God Play Dice?* Penguin Books, London.

12 Rudenski AS, Matthews DR, Levy JC *et al.* (1991) Understanding 'insulin resistance': both glucose resistance and insulin resistance are required to model human diabetes. *Metabolism.* **40**(9): 908–17.

13 Gallichan M (1997) Self monitoring of glucose by people with diabetes: evidence based practice. *BMJ.* **314**: 964–7.

14 Schaffer WM (1986) Order and chaos in ecological systems. *Ecology.* **66**(1): 93–106.

15 Glass L, Kaplan D (1993) Time series analysis of complex dynamics in physiology and medicine. *Medical Progress through Technology.* **19**(3): 115–28.

16 Kroll MH (1999) Biological variation of glucose and insulin includes a deterministic chaotic component. *Biosystems.* **50**: 189–201.

17 Riva A, Bellazzi R (1996) Learning temporal probabilistic causal models from longitudinal data. *Artificial Intelligence in Medicine.* **8**: 217–34.

18 Garfinkel A, Spano ML, Ditto W *et al.* (1992) Controlling cardiac chaos. *Science.* **257**: 1230–5.

CHAPTER 6

Complexity and mental health

Rachel A Heath

Introduction

Human behaviour in all of its forms evolves over time. This means, of course, that the most interesting features of behaviour, for both clinicians and lay people, are changes occurring from one time period to the next. These fluctuations are responsible for the variety in behaviour that characterises a person's personality as well as their general adjustment to a frequently unpredictable environment. When things go wrong, people are often sensitive to any change in the behaviour of their friends and loved ones. This calls for medical intervention in the most serious maladaptive crises.

Many behavioural disorders can change their qualitative properties quite markedly without any discernible external precedents. Such behaviour fluctuations might be generated by a gradual change in the underlying physiological, and possibly psychological, processes. Unfortunately, such endogenous bases for behaviour change are frequently overlooked in current medical practice, resulting in a possibly vain search for causal agents. In such circumstances, it may be impossible to find a reliable external cause for the client's complaint, resulting in heartache and confusion for everyone, especially the patient, professionals and family.

Diseases that exhibit dynamic variability accompanied by no obvious causal agent are termed dynamic disorders. Examples include chronic fatigue, diabetes, asthma and depression. The frequent presence of non-smooth fluctuations, such as occur when a person collapses suddenly from an asthma attack, suggests that these disorders are governed by non-linear processes. Developments in non-linear science over the past four decades suggest that apparently random behaviour can be generated from a non-linear process without added noise. Of course, in real-life non-linear systems, noise, or stochasticity, is a common accompaniment. This combination suggests the term 'stochaos', a combination of non-linear determinism (NLD), or perhaps chaos, and pure randomness. This idea is related to Freeman's proposal for brain dynamics.[1]

An interesting aspect of stochaos is the important balance between NLD and noise. In several dynamic disorders, such as depression, the extent of maladaptive behaviour increases as the NLD component starts to predominate. Normal mood fluctuations require sufficient complexity, provided perhaps by a noise source. Otherwise, such mood fluctuations become both too regular and progressively less responsive to environmental stressors.

The complex interaction between environmental influences and endogenous processes in dynamic disorders ensures that identification of causality is virtually impossible. Moreover, any qualitative change in dynamic disorders can result from the effects of both exogenous and endogenous control processes. For example, if the time course is chaotic, then either control or anti-control of chaos, techniques based on a fundamental property of chaotic systems, might have valuable applications. These include controlling epileptic seizures and alleviating brain dysfunction by direct stimulation (see Heath[2] for both the underlying theory and some illustrative examples).

This chapter begins by describing syndromes in mental health that exhibit behaviour characteristic of dynamic disorders. Then follows a comparison between normal and abnormal cases, highlighting differences in the non-linear dynamics resulting from ill health. Issues of measurement are important since most of the commonly employed monitoring procedures are ill suited for fine-grained temporal monitoring of human behaviour. Following some illustrative data analyses, future prospects for diagnosis and monitoring of mental dysfunction are proposed.

Complexity indices for physiological and psychological time series

Complexity is a very difficult concept to define precisely. This is especially the case when we are unsure as to which part of a biological process the term refers; the measurements we observe are too complicated for us to understand, and the underlying physiological or psychological processes are themselves complex. These are vexing issues about which a full understanding is yet to be achieved.

Several useful indices for quantifying the complexity of sequential data have been devised. Commonly used complexity measures include the correlation dimension, D_2, and the maximum Lyapunov exponent. Both measures require large amounts of stable data for their accurate estimation, a rare occurrence in physiological and psychological applications (see Heath[2] for details). D_2 quantifies the number of dimensions (possibly fractional) needed to represent the data fluctuations, while the maximum Lyapunov exponent measures how rapidly nearby data points change their relative locations over time. A positive Lyapunov exponent is a necessary, but not sufficient, condition for chaos. By themselves, D_2 and the Lyapunov exponent do not provide unequivocal evidence for non-linearity. For example, Shen et al.[3] have warned that low D_2 estimates can be computed from linearly transformed white noise.

One of the most frequently applied quantitative methods in physiology is approximate entropy (ApEn).[4] ApEn measures irregularity in a time series, being especially suited for analysing the kinds of short noisy series arising in medical applications. ApEn measures the likelihood that runs of data patterns that are close for several successive observations remain close at future times. Regularity in the data produces low ApEn values, whereas randomness produces large values.

Unfortunately, ApEn estimates can only be compared when the number of data points analysed is similar across conditions. In particular, ApEn is not invariant when the data are transformed, even merely to equate means and variances. Provided at least 1000 observations are used, the standard error of ApEn remains relatively small, allowing statistical comparisons between ApEn values from different conditions. As a measure of entropy, or disorder, ApEn is relatively unaffected by extreme data values. Loss of complexity, as indicated by smaller values of

ApEn, is a generic feature of pathological dynamics evidenced by lower entropy, although there are exceptions, such as in atrial fibrillation.

Recently, several new complexity measures, analogous to ApEn, have been devised. Sample entropy[5] is a variant of ApEn that is independent of sample length. A generalisation, multiscale entropy, is constant across all timescales for persistent processes, but declines monotonically with time for white noise. Multiscale entropy has been applied in cardiac physiology to distinguish between healthy heart function, congestive heart failure and atrial fibrillation.

Torres and Gamero[6] have proposed that entropy measures are more sensitive to changes in qualitative complexity of time series than is ApEn and can be computed more efficiently. Relative entropy measures are superior to ApEn in tracking changes in complexity in a heart rate (HR) series and, unlike ApEn, are relatively unaffected by superimposed noise.

Another complexity index, detrended fluctuation analysis (DFA),[7] can detect long-range correlations in time series. Such correlations are frequently observed in physiological processes that persist over time, leading to detectable correlations between activity separated by considerable temporal lags. Computational details are contained in Heath.[2] DFA provides an estimate of a scaling parameter, α, for which $\alpha = 0.5$ implies a random walk with uncorrelated increments, whereas $1 > \alpha > 0.5$ indicates long-range correlation or persistence. $0 < \alpha < 0.5$ implies anti-persistence with long and short values tending to alternate. $\alpha = 1$ corresponds to $1/f$, or pink, noise (where f is the frequency), and $\alpha = 1.5$ implies brown noise, an integrated form of a random walk. In general, the larger the value of α, the smoother the time series. For example, normal HR time series exhibit pink noise, whereas those from a diseased heart may be almost Brownian, with α equal to about 1.24. Occasionally it is worthwhile computing DFA for two different timescales – short and long. The Hurst coefficient, H, provides a measure similar to α in DFA. H equals 0.5 for a completely random process, is less than 0.5 for an anti-persistent process and is greater than 0.5 for a persistent process.

Dynamic disorders in mental health

Many mental illnesses and neurological dysfunctions are chronic disorders controlled, but not completely cured, by conventional medical and psychological interventions. Consequently they satisfy the requirements for dynamical diseases proposed by Bélair et al.[8] According to Mackay and Glass,[9] pioneers in the application of non-linear dynamics for understanding dynamic disorders, non-linear processes can be used to explain both normal and pathological behaviour. This results, perhaps, from subtle fluctuations in the parameters driving the underlying physiological process. Their proposal for more adequately understanding such processes is to first devise a mathematical or computer model, evaluate its behaviour as parameters are manipulated, and compare its output with normal and pathological function in humans. Once a model has been shown to be adequate, it can then be used for both diagnosis and treatment evaluation. However, few such models exist and more research is needed.

By considering mental disorders as dynamic complex systems, the disease process can be represented by a relatively small number of hypothetical internal variables, or parameters. Any apparent causal influences are inherent in the dynamics of the disease process itself, with potential beneficial implications for more reliable treatment and prognosis. One advantage might be that mental disorders can be categorised by similarities in their dynamics rather than by reference to specific symptom constellations. This proposal might make therapeutic agents more effective, especially those with clearly defined effects on the mechanisms responsible for the progress parameters of a dynamic disorder.

We now consider applications of non-linear dynamics in such representative mental and neurological diseases as bipolar disorder, chronic depression, Parkinson's disease, schizophrenia, migraine headache and epilepsy. Brief comments on the dynamics observed in panic and anxiety disorders are also provided.

Gottschalk et al.[10] conducted a pioneering dynamic analysis of bipolar disorder. It had been assumed that mood fluctuations in bipolar disorder were governed by multiples of an approximately 48-hour cycle, with rapid cycling being a risk for long-term sufferers. Gottschalk et al. selected as their experimental group rapid-cycling patients satisfying the DSM criteria for bipolar disorder, who had experienced at least four mood-changing episodes in the previous 12 months.

Each patient and their matched control maintained a daily mood diary by placing a cross on a scale ranging from 'best I ever felt' at one end to 'worst I ever felt' at the other end. Mood ratings were obtained over a period ranging from one to two and a half years, yielding time series with approximately 700 observations. The data were analysed using both linear and non-linear analysis methods. For example, the linear power spectrum depicted the relative predominance (power) of each mood fluctuation frequency. For these data, the power spectrum was linear with a negative slope when both the power and frequency scales were logarithmically transformed. This slope was -1.29 for the bipolar patients and almost exactly half in absolute terms (-0.69) for the controls. Since lower slopes indicate noisier mood fluctuations, it is possible that bipolar patients display insufficient noise in their mood fluctuations, a dynamic indicator of abnormality. Such linear log–log spectra imply that mood fluctuations are timescale invariant, suggesting that equally diagnostic results might apply when mood ratings are observed at considerably shorter time intervals.

Whereas the number of degrees of freedom required to accommodate mood fluctuations for bipolar patients was less than four, as indicated by a D_2 estimate of 3.2, that for control subjects was virtually unbounded. This result suggests a lower complexity of mood expression for bipolar clients. By plotting successive mood ratings against each other, the resulting 'phase plots' for bipolar clients were uniformly more highly structured than those for the controls (except for one bipolar client who had responded well to treatment). Gottschalk et al. proposed that the different dynamics exhibited by bipolar and control clients result from differences in how any coupling between endogenous and environmental influences affects mood dynamics.[10] When the characteristic mood fluctuation is chaotic in distressed people, anti-control of chaos might be used to redirect the dynamics from the chaotic regime towards a more complex, random process.[11] Perhaps electroconvulsive therapy achieves an analogous effect by injecting sufficient neural noise to restore normal mood fluctuations in chronic depression.

In a similar study, Woyshville et al.[12] obtained 90 daily mood ratings on a visual analog scale from 36 patients suffering from affective instability and from 27 control subjects. The log–log spectrum slope was -0.43 for patients and -0.22 for controls, a similar ratio to that obtained by Gottschalk et al.[10] Perhaps the ratio of exponents from healthy and unhealthy people may be compared in different situations, but their exact values may rely on the rating method used.

More recently, Heiby et al.[13] studied mood fluctuation dynamics in two young women, one with chronic depression and the other with no history of depression. Supportive psychotherapy over the past three years had had no effect on depressive episode frequency for the depressed client. Depression/sadness, as measured by a Likert rating scale, was regularly calibrated using a telephone version of the Beck Depression Inventory,[14] yielding 80% agreement. The participants rated their mood every hour for 10 hours a day for six months, prompted by a watch alarm.

The control subject provided 1840 data points (2% missing), a similar number (4.4% missing) being obtained for the depressed subject. This number of data points is sufficient to apply basic methods for non-linear data analysis, provided the system has fewer than four degrees of freedom.[15]

The depression ratings were significantly higher for the depressed subject, with some evidence for persistence of mood. The control subject exhibited anti-persistence of mood fluctuations, leading to greater mood variability. Heiby et al.[13] proposed the maladaptive determinism hypothesis under which the diseased state is characterised by a greater proportion of deterministic, or more predictable, behaviour than occurs for healthy individuals. The greater the determinism, the less likely the individual can adjust to the added complexity of environmental demands. So clinical assessment must examine the properties of mood fluctuations as well as the static level of dysfunction, as measured at a single point in time using questionnaires such as the Beck Depression Inventory.

Spectral analysis of the two clients' data revealed significant periodicities, probably resulting from menstrual cycle effects, of 26 days for the depressed and 23 days for the non-depressed woman. This periodicity was removed from each power spectrum prior to further data analyses. The log–log power spectrum slope was -1.95 for the non-depressed subject and -2.15 for the depressed subject. Although these values are in the same direction as those observed by Gottschalk et al.[10] they are much larger and lie in a range characteristic of brown noise.

D_2 was 2.7 for the depressed subject and essentially unbounded for the non-depressed control. Support for the maladaptive determinism hypothesis was obtained by showing that this complexity value was significantly less than the 4.0 computed for a comparison time series that had the same linear properties as the data, but no non-linearity.

Mood ratings suffer from subjective influences and measurement difficulties, it being difficult for raters to maintain consistent mood estimates over extended time periods. Furthermore, the ordinal scale frequently used in mood rating cannot always be analysed legitimately using the available quantitative techniques (but see Gregson[16] and Gregson and Leahan[17] for some new techniques).

Since it is difficult to acquire sufficient mood ratings to apply the most sensitive of non-linear techniques, physiological correlates such as heart rate are attractive alternatives. Major depression produces decreased cardiac vagal function, together with a relative increase in sympathetic activity, and the associated heart disease risk increases by a factor of between 2 and 5. There is also an increased risk of stroke. Depression is related to decreased HR variability in coronary heart disease.[18]

Earlier research had shown that a non-linear measure based on symbolic dynamics, a procedure that transforms continuous HR into a sequence of discrete symbols, is the best discriminator between those with panic disorder and controls.

These patients also have a significantly lower maximum Lyapunov exponent than suitably matched controls. A similar finding occurred for children with anxiety disorder, with non-linear parameters being diagnostic, whereas the linear spectral components did not discriminate between this group and a control group.[18]

Yeragani et al.[18] measured HR in 18 age-matched control subjects and 14 patients with major depressive disorder. Rosenstein's method was used to compute the largest Lyapunov exponent.[19] The statistics of extreme values of the HR time series were also used to determine whether the series is deterministic or random. The largest Lyapunov exponent was significantly lower in patients than controls, as was the ratio of Lyapunov exponents computed for low-frequency (0.04–0.15 Hz) versus high-frequency (0.15–0.50 Hz) HR spectral components.

So depressed patients exhibited lower HR complexity, resulting in a higher level of sympathetic activity than was observed in the controls. Yeragani et al.[18] suggest that treating depression using cognitive behavioural therapy may increase HR variability and so provide some relief from the physiological, as well as the psychological, correlates of depression.

Heart rate has been analysed using non-linear procedures, showing, for example, that a decrease in complexity with heart disease is similar in principle to the decrease in complexity for mood rating data in depression. For example, Zbilut et al.[20] have shown how recurrence quantification analysis (RQA), a relatively simple procedure for examining both the qualitative and quantitative features of time-series data, can be used to discriminate between control and diseased states using HR data.

Rao and Yeragani[21] used RQA to investigate variations in HR dynamics for patients with panic disorder. When compared with age-matched controls, people suffering from panic disorder exhibited a less complex and more predictable HR signal. This finding suggests that HR can be represented primarily by a non-linear process for the patients but that a more noisy representation is required for the controls.

The motor tremor that characterises Parkinson's disease also tends to be more organised and possibly chaotic when compared with the noisier tremor observed in age-controlled normals.[22] This provides another example of maladaptive determinism, this time in psychomotor control.

Non-linear methods have been used to investigate functional differences between clients with schizophrenia and their matched controls. Clients with schizophrenia seem to respond in a two-choice decision-making task with less complex response sequences than controls.[23] Dünki et al.[24] examined the dynamics of the change from one mental state (psychosis) to another (non-psychosis) in schizophrenia. Non-psychosis is related to a laminar, or steady-state, phase, whereas psychosis reflects a turbulent phase of a disorder. Such a rapid change from steady-state behaviour to psychosis involves a threshold, or 'bifurcation'. The relatively sudden change in dynamics resulting from a bifurcation occurs when the parameters driving a non-linear dynamical system exceed specific values. (See also p. 56.)

In the Dünki et al. study,[24] fluctuations in psychotic symptoms in clients with schizophrenia were rated on a seven-point Likert scale, ranging from 'relaxed and balanced' (1) to 'hallucinations, catatonic behaviour' (7). Ratings higher than 3, 'strong withdrawal or aggressive', were regarded as psychotic. The slope of the log–log power spectrum for a typical patient with schizophrenia was −0.87, indicating more noise than was observed for manic depressive patients by Gottschalk et al.[10]

According to Paulus and Braff,[25] an altered sequential or temporal architecture serves as a basic deficiency in schizophrenia. The disease dynamics consist of bursts of complex non-linear phenomena interspersed with random events, probably resulting in the disturbance of associations, a characteristic feature of schizophrenia. Overstimulation, or sensory overload, leads to fixity or even catatonia, suggesting that behavioural output is not proportional to stimulus input, a characteristic property of non-linear complex systems.

In schizophrenia, healthy flexible behaviour and unhealthy fixated behaviour exist at various times in the same patient. As Paulus et al.[23] found, some, but not all, patients generate choice sequences that are highly predictable. At other times such sequences are highly unpredictable, implying intermittent behaviour dynamics. Such behaviour occurs during the patient's first psychotic episode and appears to be fairly stable over time. The intermittent behaviour is related to activation of the prefrontal-parietal cortex, as has been verified by brain imaging studies. Time series generated by intermittent behaviour have high variability, are highly sensitive to perturbations and contain complex temporal correlations. Treatment methods for schizophrenia might profitably remove or minimise the effects of intermittency on cognitive processing.

Kirsch et al.[26] have suggested that patients with schizophrenia tend to exhibit higher dimensional complexity for both involved tasks and control conditions. The higher values occur mainly at frontal electrode sites, with decreased dimensional complexity being observed for central sites. Subjects with schizophrenia perform more poorly than controls on continuous performance tasks (CPT), such as the AX task which requires subjects to respond to the letter X only when it is preceded by an A.

Eighty-seven patients and 30 controls, matched for age and gender, participated in the experiment. In the AX task, 180 stimuli were presented for 100 ms each, 30 of them being targets. A second task (concept change, CC) involved detecting changes in the categories from which nouns were sampled. There were 90 stimuli presented for 500 ms each, with 30 of them being targets. EEG was recorded from one site, C_z.

The patients produced significantly more omission errors on both the AX and CC tasks than controls, the mean response time being significantly longer for the group with schizophrenia in both tasks. The correlation dimension, D_2, tended to be larger for the subjects with schizophrenia in both tasks, but the mean values were high for all subjects with values exceeding 10.0, signifying noise rather than determinism. Differences in D_2 were only significant for a period of one and two minutes following task commencement. The increase in dimensional complexity for subjects with schizophrenia may result from the extra difficulty of the tasks for these people, or else there is more noise in their EEG data irrespective of the task difficulty, the more likely explanation given the high D_2 values.

The migraine headache is a functional neurological disorder with disturbed autoregulation of cerebral blood flow. West et al. (2003)[27] have suggested that cerebral blood flow is multifractal, a process with complex dynamics in several distinct dimensions. West et al. showed that middle cerebral artery flow velocity is multifractal with a wide range of fractal values for normals but with a much restricted fractal range for migraine sufferers. Since multifractal processes are highly adaptive, a migraine headache leads to a less adaptive, and less complex, cerebral blood-flow pattern.

Epilepsy affects 1% of the general population and 25% of cases do not respond readily to medical interventions. Furthermore, the occurrence of epileptic seizures is fundamentally unpredictable.[28] Epilepsy also produces low-dimensional and therefore less complex brain activity, so that recovery from a seizure results in a reversion to more noisy, and therefore more complex, brain dynamics.[29]

In a typical epileptic episode, the ictal stage occurs at seizure onset and is characterised by high-amplitude, organised and self-sustained rhythmic electrical discharges; the postictal stage is the period between seizure and normal brain activity; finally, the interictal stage occurring between the postictal stage of one seizure and the preictal stage of another, is characterised by sharp waves and spikes. Seizures may represent a reset of the brain from order back into chaos. Positive Lyapunov exponents tend to be lower during the ictal stage, indicating lower complexity and greater predictability. However, as Gregson and Leahan[17] have emphasised, it is difficult to extract non-linear indices from short time series that are not low dimensional, that are not stationary and that are contaminated by noise. Using RQA recurrence plots, a decrease in percentage determinism (%DET) occurs about 15 seconds before the seizure,[30] suggesting that a loss of complexity may serve as a warning signal for an ensuing seizure.

Diambraa et al.[31] used ApEn to identify epileptic seizures in EEG data. The participants were ten normal males in the awake condition with eyes closed, who served as controls, as well as eight epileptic patients, two female and six male. A sliding window of 220 EEG observations (about one second) provided the time series for data analysis. A decrease in ApEn during the ictal period suggested that synchronous discharge during a seizure led to a loss of signal complexity. There was a sudden decrease in ApEn around seizure onset, with mean ApEn during a seizure being 0.34 for the patients with epilepsy compared with a value of 0.75 for the controls, at a comparable time. Since ApEn can be computed using relatively short EEG samples, the lack of stationarity of the EEG signal is not quite so critical.

Non-linear analyses of data acquired from a variety of neurological and psychiatric illnesses support the maladaptive determinism hypothesis,[13] illness being characterised by less complex dynamics. This finding was obtained using both physiological (HR, EEG) and psychological (behaviour rating) data. In the next section, we examine evidence for analogous results in ageing. In this case, the proposition that ageing is associated with a loss of complexity is not supported in all applications.

Brain complexity, disease and ageing

As the brain loses efficiency with age, brain function complexity might decrease correspondingly. However, Anokhin et al.[32] found that the predictability of EEG signals decreased with age, implying that brain activity becomes more complex. However, this finding may result from an increase in brain noise with age, leading to an illusory increase in complexity.

Pikkujamsu et al.[33] obtained 24-hour ECG recordings with healthy subjects whose age ranged from 1 to 82 years. From middle to old age there was a linear decrease in ApEn, as well as in the power-law exponent (-1.15 to -1.38), but an increase in DFA slope relative to the values obtained for children and young adults. These results imply a loss in heart function complexity with increasing age, in contrast to the increase obtained by Anokhin *et al.* for EEG.

Vaillancourt and Newell[34] have reviewed changes in complexity with age in various physiological and psychological disorders. Complexity in a standing posture task, as measured by ApEn, increased from 5-year-olds to young adults and then declined thereafter with age. Similar results occur in motor tremor, as indicated by a reduction in tremor complexity during the age-dependent time course in Parkinson's disease (PD). A progressive decrease in complexity as disease state worsens was indicated by a significant negative correlation between ApEn and PD severity rating ($r = -0.84$).

Elderly subjects have reduced HR complexity, the complexity decreasing steadily with age for people over 40. HR complexity is lower in patients with diabetes than for controls. Infants at risk for sudden infant death syndrome, and heart transplant patients also exhibit lower HR complexity. EEG complexity decreases with age and with the neuropathy that occurs during the early stages of Alzheimer's disease.[34]

Not all diseases are associated with lower dynamic complexity. There is less correlated structure (less predictability) in the gait of Huntington's disease patients when compared with controls. In agromegaly, there is an increase in the complexity of growth hormone dynamics. Also, leutinising hormone (LH) and testosterone time series are more complex in the elderly than in young people. In Cushing's disease, adrenocorticotropin (ACTH) and cortisol hormone time series are more complex, as indicated by higher ApEn measures, than those observed in controls.[34]

However Goldberger *et al.*[35] have warned about the indiscriminant use of such measures to indicate changes in complexity. For example, ApEn is a regularity statistic, not really a measure of complexity. It does not probe non-linearity nor does it quantify fractal scaling behaviour, so an increase in regularity does not imply decreased complexity. A breakdown of long-range correlations in physiological systems can lead to highly periodic behaviour, a random walk or completely unpredictable white noise. So complexity loss can also result from a breakdown in long-range correlations. These technical issues need to be considered when associating the disease state or ageing with the complexity of the underlying physiological or psychological system dynamics.

Conclusions

We have seen how concepts from non-linear dynamics can elucidate the time course of illness in diverse areas of mental health. In all cases, a variety of qualitative and quantitative measures can reveal interesting differences between healthy and unhealthy states, provided that sufficient sequentially recorded data are available for analysis. It is not always the case that disease and ageing lead to less complex dynamics, but this situation seems to apply to depression in particular. The large differences between the dynamics revealed by individual patients, as well as the measurement difficulties arising from noisy and highly non-stationary physiological processes, ensure that any assessment of complexity in mental health applications is itself a complicated process.

Perhaps the most useful application of non-linear dynamics and complexity theory in mental health is in providing a novel technology for classifying mental illnesses and for offering possibly useful interventions, both pharmaceutically and behaviourally, once the dynamics of the illness have been understood. Rather than only identifying the symptoms presented at any point in time, this technology will provide guidelines for new classifications of mental illnesses based on dynamic time-dependent processes, as well as offering new applications for current and future medications. The effectiveness of clinical interventions will be determined by their ability to alter the dynamics of the disorder so that a more adaptive response to environmental and intrinsic stressors can occur.

References

1   Freeman WJ (2000) A proposed name for aperiodic brain activity: stochastic chaos. *Neural Networks.* **13**: 11–13.
2   Heath RA (2000) *Nonlinear Dynamics: techniques and applications in psychology.* Lawrence Erlbaum and Assoc, Mahwah, NJ.
3   Shen Y, Olbrich E, Achermann P *et al.* (2003) Dimensional complexity and spectral properties of the human sleep EEG. *Clinical Neurophysiology.* **114**: 199–209.
4   Pincus S (1995) Approximate entropy (ApEn) as a complexity measure. *Chaos.* **5**: 110–17.
5   Costa M, Goldberger AL, Peng C-K (2002) Multiscale entropy analysis of complex physiologic time series. *Physical Review Letters.* **89**: 068102.
6   Torres ME, Gamero LG (2000) Relative complexity changes in time series using information measures. *Physica A.* **286**: 457–73.
7   Peng C-K, Havlin S, Stanley HE *et al.* (1995). Quantification of scaling exponents and crossover phenomena in nonstationary heartbeat time series. *Chaos.* **5**: 82–7.
8   Bélair J, Glass L, van der Heiden U *et al.* (1995) *Dynamical Disease: mathematical analysis of human illness.* American Institute of Physics, Woodbury, NY.
9   Mackay MC, Glass L (1977) Oscillation and chaos in physiological control systems. *Science.* **197**: 287–9.
10 Gottschalk A, Bauer MS, Whybrow PC (1995) Evidence of chaotic mood variation in bipolar disorder. *Archives of General Psychiatry.* **52**: 947–59.
11 Schiff SJ, Jerger K, Duong DH *et al.* (1994) Controlling chaos in the brain. *Nature.* **370**: 615–20.
12 Woyshville MJ, Lackamp JM, Eisengart JA *et al.* (1999) On the meaning and measurement of affective instability: clues from chaos theory. *Biological Psychiatry.* **45**: 261–9.
13 Heiby EM, Pagano IS, Blaine DD *et al.* (2003) Modelling unipolar depression as a chaotic process. *Psychological Assessment.* **15**: 426–34.
14 Beck AT (1967) *Depression: clinical, experimental, and theoretical aspects.* Hoeber, New York.
15 Heath RA, Kelly A, Longstaff M (2000) Detecting nonlinearity in psychological data: techniques and applications. *Behavior Research Methods, Instrumentation and Computers.* **32**: 280–9.

16 Gregson RAM (2002) Scaling quasi-periodic psychological functions. *Behaviormetrika.* **29**: 41–57.

17 Gregson RAM, Leahan K (2003) Forcing function effects on nonlinear trajectories: identifying very local brain dynamics. *Nonlinear Dynamics, Psychology, and Life Sciences.* **7**: 139–59.

18 Yeragani VK, Krishna Rao KAR, Smitha MR *et al.* (2002) Diminished chaos of heart rate time series in patients with major depression. *Biological Psychiatry.* **51**: 733–44.

19 Rosenstein MT, Collins JJ, De Luca CJ (1993) A practical method for calculating largest Lyapunov exponents from small data sets. *Physica D.* **65**: 117–34.

20 Zbilut JP, Webber CL, Zak M (1998) Quantification of heart rate variability using methods derived from nonlinear dynamics. In: GM Drzewiecki, J K-J Li (eds) *Analysis and Assessment of Cardiovascular Function*, pp. 324–34. Springer-Verlag, New York.

21 Rao RKA, Yeragani VK (2001) Decreased chaos and increased nonlinearity of heart rate time series in patients with panic disorder. *Autonomic Neuroscience: Basic and Clinical.* **88**: 99–108.

22 Gantert C, Honerkamp J, Timmer J (1992) Analyzing the dynamics of hand tremor time series. *Biological Cybernetics.* **66**: 479–84.

23 Paulus MP, Geyer MA, Braff DL (1996) Use of methods from chaos theory to quantify a fundamental dysfunction in the behavioral organisation of schizophrenic patients. *American Journal of Psychiatry.* **153**: 714–17.

24 Dünki RM, Kellerb E, Meiera PF *et al.* (2000) Temporal patterns of human behaviour: are there signs of deterministic $1/f$ scaling? *Physica A.* **276**: 596–609.

25 Paulus MP, Braff DL (2003) Chaos and schizophrenia: does the method fit the madness? *Biological Psychiatry.* **53**: 3–11.

26 Kirsch UP, Besthorn C, Klein S *et al.* (2000) The dimensional complexity of the EEG during cognitive tasks reflects the impaired information processing in schizophrenic patients. *International Journal of Psychophysiology.* **36**: 237–46.

27 West BJ, Latka M, Glaubic-Latka M, Latka D (2003) Multifractality of cerebral blood flow. *Physica A.* **318**: 453–60.

28 Pardalos PM, Yatsenko V, Sackellares JC *et al.* (2003) Analysis of EEG data using optimization, statistics, and dynamical system techniques. *Computational Statistics and Data Analysis.* **43**: 79–108.

29 Andrzejak RG, Widman G, Lehnertz K *et al.* (2001) The epileptic process as nonlinear deterministic dynamics in a stochastic environment: an evaluation on medial temporal lobe epilepsy. *Epilepsy Research.* **44**: 129–40.

30 Thomasson N, Hoeppner TJ, Webber CL *et al.* (2001) Recurrence quantification in epileptic EEGs. *Physics Letters A.* **279**: 94–101.

31 Diambraa L, Bastos de Figueiredo JC, Malta CP (1999) Epileptic activity recognition in EEG recording. *Physica A.* **273**: 495–505.

32 Anokhin AP, Birbaumer N, Lutzenberger W *et al.* (1996) Age increases brain complexity. *Electroencephalography and Clinical Neurophysiology.* **99**: 63–8.

33 Pikkujamsu SM, Makikallio TH, Sourander LB *et al.* (1999) Cardiac interbeat interval dynamics from childhood to senescence: comparison of conventional and new measures based on fractals and chaos theory. *Circulation.* **100**: 393–9.

34 Vaillancourt DE, Newell KM (2002) Changing complexity in human behavior and physiology through aging and disease. *Neurobiology of Aging*. **23**: 1–11.

35 Goldberger AL, Peng C-K, Lipsitz LA (2002) What is physiologic complexity and how does it change with aging and disease? *Neurobiology of Aging*. **23**: 23–6.

PART THREE

Health informatics and the delivery of clinical care

CHAPTER 7

Decision support, complexity and primary healthcare

Paul Robinson

This chapter is about the way evidence-based guidance is represented in the decision-making process in the primary care consultation. The key message is that 'failure' to follow published guidance is often not down to lack of awareness: rather, guidance is one of a number of competing voices in the consultation. Consequently, a 'simplex' approach of pushing the guidance at practitioners with more force may not be successful.

Decision making

Academic study of decision making considers three aspects:

1 *Descriptive*, i.e. how people actually do make decisions in real life.
2 *Normative*, i.e. the processes that would constitute rational decision making: what *should* happen.
3 *Prescriptive*, i.e. tools that will encourage rational action in real life: moving the descriptive towards the normative.

As Bazerman[1] suggests, exploration of the descriptive field raises awareness of bias. This realisation has prompted the desire to base decisions on rational grounds. In rational terms, a 'good' decision is not necessarily one that produces the right outcome, but is one that is made on the basis of an objective assessment of as many relevant factors as possible. Contributions to this grail of rationality and objectivity are frame analysis and structured decision aids such as decision and utility trees, SMART (**s**imple **m**ulti-**a**ttribute **r**ating **t**echnique)[2] and scenario planning.

This desire for objectivity and rationality pervades the study of medical decision making.

The medical consultation has been used as material for studying decision making,[3] the structures of professional knowledge,[4] reflective practice[5] and professional competence.[6] This interest is continued in the information age, and medicine currently provides a forum for the development of computer systems that provide information support and decision support for practitioners.[7]

Medicine is seen as a high-status profession, and medical specialism is sometimes presented as the epitome of expertise. At the same time, 'seeing the doctor' is a commonplace with which researchers and others can easily identify. The consultation is a very rich source of material. In decision-making terms, there are two main areas of decision relating to diagnosis and treatment respectively. The boundary between these two categories is often blurred, particularly in primary care, and the consultation may be represented as a single decision: 'how should I manage this case?' On the other hand, the interaction between doctor and patient can be represented as a series of scores of micro-decisions: 'should I ask this question now?'; 'should I examine this system now?'; 'should I explain what I'm doing, or just get on with it?' The communication skills aspects of the consultation have been studied in great detail.[8] Each utterance by the doctor can be interpreted as a speech act[9] or a response,[10] the consequence of which has to be considered and deliberated.

An ambiguity is the clash between medicine as scientific and medicine as humanitarian.[11] On the one hand, there is an evidence-based culture,[12] which seeks to reduce variations in practice and to promote definitions of best practice that are founded on the best available research evidence, often taken from large studies on populations. On the other, there is still a premium placed on judgement and experience and on the concept of the patient as an individual, with individual needs and an individual story. The study of narrative[13] has become identified with this latter viewpoint.

The consultation is thus a busy place, in which a number of conflicts are played out. Muir Gray[14] has proposed a model of evidence-based decision making in his document on the strategy of the National electronic Library for Health (NeLH). The NeLH is part of the Department of Health's modernisation strategy and is intended to provide access (for practitioners and patients) to the burgeoning amount of health information available. The model is shown in Figure 7.1. In this context 'evidence' is a synonym for 'guideline'.

Examples of decision support in medicine occurring in the diagnostic arena include Isabel (a Web-based paediatric service)[15] Dermis (provided in the UK as an add-on to a clinical system)[16] and scoring systems such as the HAD[17] for depression.

Therapeutic and clinical management support is provided by guidelines such as Prodigy, which is available online[18] or in book form,[19] and algorithms such as the British Thoracic Society's stepped guidance for asthma treatment.[20]

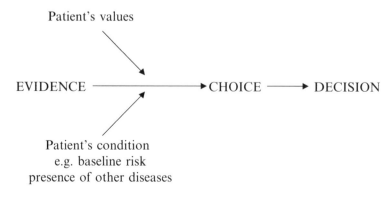

Figure 7.1 Evidence-based decision-making.

Complexity in individuals and healthcare systems

Stacey[21] has recently questioned the notion of the complex adaptive system and suggested replacing it with 'complex responsive processes'. In this chapter, I work with the idea that complexity produces emergent properties in a system that cannot be predicted by analysis of the component parts of the system. Also, taking a lead from Etienne Wenger, I suggest that the question of whether something *is* a complex system is less useful than the question 'does it help to think about this *as* a complex system?'

Recent developments in neuroscience and theories of consciousness make it perhaps easier to justify the view of individual consciousness as being an emergent property of a complex system. Ever since Descartes separated mind from body it has been natural to think of the conscious entity of an individual as a passive observer of mental function. Dennett[24,25] describes this notion as the 'Cartesian theatre', and Cohen and Stewart[26] as the 'homunculus problem': where in the homunculus does consciousness reside? Modern techniques of brain imaging are giving rise to a new notion of perception and consciousness. They have overturned the neuroscience of 20 or 30 years ago. The conclusion is that consciousness is constructed from extensive neural activity in diverse parts of the brain. It is a distributed phenomenon of the neural network, active rather than passive. Further, the generation of consciousness takes time: conscious awareness lags about 0.3–0.5 s behind events.[27]

This half-second time lag has profound implications for our understanding of how our bodies and minds work. Visual perception used to be thought of as a largely passive process, with light being transformed into neural signals in the retina and then projected to specific areas of the cerebral cortex, which 'saw' the object. The new techniques of brain imaging show that large and diverse areas of the cerebral cortex are active when an object is seen, that a mixture of 'sensory' and 'motor' areas are involved in perception, and that the subject does not become aware of seeing the object for about half a second, although the alterations in brain activity begin straight away. This leads to two questions: 'what is happening during that half-second interval?' and 'how can people play fast ball-sports?'

We will deal with the second question first. The problem arises because in games like tennis, for example, the trajectory of the ball when served by a top player lasts less than 0.3 s. Yet, frequently, the receiver of service not only manages to get racquet to ball to make a return, he or she is also able to do this in a purposeful way. In cricket, the batsman facing a fast bowler performs a similar feat. In fact, any quick reaction has the same basis, the player's body responds appropriately to the ball before the mind has had time to assemble a conscious image of it. This may explain the relative incoherence of footballers when asked to describe a goal they just scored, and how much more easily they can do the commentary after seeing a video replay.

Either top sportsmen become very good at guessing and predicting the future, or their bodies (after much training and practice) become able to respond 'automatically' to the stimulus. Neural pathways have been found that connect visual and motor systems in the thalamus, without reference to the cerebral cortex. The response time of this circuitry is much quicker (about 0.1 s), so it can account for the sportsman's quick reaction. Of course, this raises the question of how much of our normal day-to-day behaviour is 'automatic' in the same way. The idea that our language-based conscious awareness is somehow in charge and making moment-to-moment decisions becomes questionable[28].

This uncertainty is deepened by experiments on simple decision making.[29] Subjects are attached to magnetoencephalography (MEG) monitors, which record the timing of brain activity very accurately. They are asked to press a button on the arm of their chair, but can choose to do this whenever they like. The monitors again show a time lapse of 0.3–0.5 s, but in this case the time elapses from the start of the discernible change in cerebral activity to the moment when the subject is aware of making the decision to press the button. Consciousness is again lagging behind events. Who is doing the deciding?

In his book *Consciousness Explained*,[24] Daniel Dennett has explored this problem in detail, using the notion of *demons*. The term 'daemon' is used in computer programming to refer to self-contained subroutines that each look after a small part of a computer's working. The computer's operating system consists of a large number of daemons that successfully co-exist. In behavioural terms, Dennett's demons are small subunits of activity; at any point there are several available, but only one will be 'selected' and determine behaviour. This selection is, according to Dennett, a form of natural selection and not a deliberate choice of 'mind'.

For example, think of someone seeing a yellow object rolling across the floor. In size and shape and colour this could be a tennis ball or a ball of wool. Depending on the context (environment), one of these will be a better fit. In an indoor sports centre the individual will consciously see a tennis ball, in their aunt's back room he or she would see a ball of wool. Dennett's contribution is to think of individual concepts, or actions, as entities that are subject to natural selection within the brain.

Edelman and Tononi[30] come to a similar conclusion with their theory of how consciousness is generated in the brain. They suggest that for a perception or an idea to become conscious, the cluster of neuronal activity that represents it has to have sufficient energy to impinge on the dynamic core of cerebral activity. Whereas Dennett's approach is philosophical, theirs is neurobiological. Both refer in depth to Darwin and natural selection.

To many of us, this approach and this application of the familiar idea of natural selection is deeply counter-intuitive. Our world-view, and much of our morality, is based on the idea of deliberate decision making and free choice. By this we mean deliberate decision making by the 'I' that is represented by the inner voice. The way the findings of contemporary neuroscience are being interpreted suggests that the inner voice, our conscious story, is a 'remembered present',[30] an emergent construct that is a half-second behind the action, and the product not of design but of natural selection among individual elements of which we are not consciously aware. 'Mind first' is wrong, even in the realm of the mind.

Of course, no ideas are totally new, nor isolated. Dennett's daemons are reminiscent of schema theory as developed by Piaget and Bartlett.[31] The whole notion of experiential learning as developed by Dewey[32] and Kolb,[33] for example, sits easily here. More recently Richard Dawkins, writing from a Darwinist viewpoint, developed the idea of 'memes', and this torch has been carried further by others, such as Susan Blackmore.[34] Whereas Dennett is writing about the natural selection of concepts and perceptions within an individual's head, meme theory considers concepts and ideas as agents subject to natural selection in the social environment.

Voices and subcultural language in the consultation

Some years ago I embarked on a research project that looked at knowledge use in the GP consultation.[11] As a medical teacher I was struck by the difference between the formal knowledge that I was taught in my own training and the knowledge that I actually used when working with patients. The idea behind the study was to describe and classify the knowledge used by GPs in day-to-day work. Data were collected in the form of transcripts of consultations and of qualitative interviews with the GPs. This was analysed using a grounded theory methodology.

The pattern that emerged from this analysis typified knowledge primarily by its source rather than its type. Whereas formal classifications of knowledge make a distinction between prepositional knowledge and impression or experience, for example, it was never possible to make these theoretical constructs, which are based on epistemology, fit the data. The model that emerged is summarised in Figure 7.2.

Up to 170 knowledge items could be identified in a 10-minute consultation. The knowledge used in the consultation could be mapped out according to the four categories outlined in Figure 7.2, with the practitioner accessing knowledge from different sources in turn.

Table 7.1 shows how, in a routine consultation, the GP is using knowledge gained from different sources. All this information is available in the consultation, either from the patient or from the GP's memory. This is the traditional view of the expert–client relationship: the expert acquires knowledge through initial training, experience and continual professional development, and then dispenses this knowledge to the client.

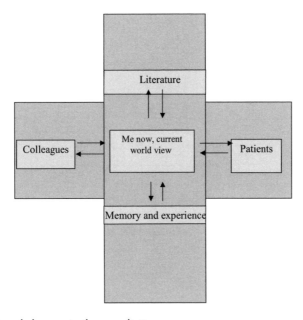

Figure 7.2 Knowledge use in the consultation.

Table 7.1 Knowledge flow in part of a consultation for cystitis

Patient	Memory/experience	Colleagues	Literature
This woman has blood in her urine, and it burns when she passes urine			These are symptoms of cystitis, which is common. Blood in urine can indicate serious conditions
She had a similar episode last year, which settled with antibiotics			
	Some people are very worried when they see blood in their urine		
She does not look worried			
			Nitrites in the urine strongly suggest infection
She has ++ nitrites		We normally check MSU in every suspected case of urine infection	
		Practice policy is to use a 5-day course of trimethoprim	Three-day course of trimethoprim is usually sufficient treatment for cystitis
	I can remember failure of treatment with a 3-day course		

Most of the time the expert's knowledge and experience are sufficient. If not, then the four different sources of knowledge can be consulted: the GP can ask a colleague (either another GP or a specialist), go to textbooks or journals, or look at the notes of another patient with a similar problem. Expertise is deployed in the choice of knowledge source and the way in which it is accessed and then interpreted.

Voices

The model shown in Figure 7.2 is based on practice. It is a description of where the practitioner 'goes' to find things out. A key feature of the model is illustrated by the bi-directional arrows. In the interaction with the patient, for example, the doctor is affecting the patient as much as the patient is affecting the doctor. Similarly, while the doctor is drawing from the literature and using it as a knowledge source, he or she is also contributing to it by virtue of the clinical records made.

The work of Vygotsky and Bahktin, as described by Wertsch,[35] provides another perspective on this. Vygotsky and Bahktin were contemporaries in the Soviet Union, working from Marxist principles in the early part of the twentieth century. They developed a socio-cultural approach to learning and action. Vygotsky's notion of the *zone of proximal development* described how cognition and learning are socially distributed, and the way in which learning can take place in conversation between two individuals and how it is then impossible to say who is learner and who is teacher, since neither may have had the knowledge before the conversation started. He also viewed an individual's learning as an internalising of conversations and social activity. His point was that learning takes place in the social milieu first, and later becomes set in the individual. There are obvious parallels here with Dewey's, and later Kolb's, work on experiential learning; their emphasis is on experience of the individual rather than the social group. Finally, Vygotsky describes how inner speech is a sense-making phenomenon: sense being a dynamic and context-related thing as opposed to dictionary-based meanings, which are static and abstract.

Bahktin's contribution is to think of utterances of an individual, first as a response to someone else. Second, he describes the concept of *multivoicedness*. Since an individual's thoughts are developed by internalising conversations with others, any utterance made by an individual contains elements of another's voice. So there are always at least two voices in play at any time. This idea is developed by showing how parody, sarcasm and ventriloquism are ways that people introduce other voices in their speech for particular purposes of emphasis, humour and so on. Third, he describes how social languages develop within a national language. Meanings vary within a single mother tongue, depending on the social context and the sense making that goes on in conversations within a community.

What has this got to do with decision support?

On one level, further analysis of transcripts of GP consultations from this perspective throws up numerous examples of different voices in the utterances of a single practitioner. In our context, they can be related to the sources of knowledge shown in Figure 7.2. At different times a practitioner will invoke another voice using formal guidelines: 'look, it says here ...'; or colleagues: 'no sensible GP is going to ...'; or other patients: 'most people find ...' to support a course of action.

At another level, the heterogeneity of voices that is available to one individual creates another set of 'choices': in which voice does the person speak in a particular context? It may be useful to think of voices as entities that are subject to the rules of natural selection, to think of utterances as emerging from a melee of competing possible options.

From these perspectives, the task for decision support is much more than just to deliver factually correct advice to the point of work. It must also be appropriate in terms of the social context and the subcultural languages that are available to the practitioner.

Levels of analysis: a view from political science

A political approach to context is provided by political scientist Rick Wylie. He originally developed these ideas in relation to environmental issues (personal communication), but they transfer easily to health.

'Levels of analysis' is a way of looking at things that is commonly used in political science. The basic thesis is that people apply different values depending on what level of analysis they are working at. Politically, this can be represented as macro (corresponding roughly to the national and policy level), meso (corresponding to a regional or locality level and systems to implement policy) and micro (corresponding to individuals' actions and choices).

One example is the way that people think about environmental disaster. If asked how much should be spent to clean up after an oil spill, they will quote figures in millions that would translate to several dollars per head. Asked how much they would be prepared to contribute, the figure is normally in cents.

Moving this into the medical field, take the instance of antibiotic prescribing for respiratory infections. Considerations at the macro level are with the overall effect of antibiotic prescribing: drug costs, use of GPs' time (unnecessary appointments), side effects and antibiotic resistance. This generates a policy of reducing antibiotic prescribing, which is implemented at the meso level by systems such as audit, monitoring of prescribing, visits by pharmaceutical advisors. At the micro level the GP considers the expectations of the patient, the likely risk of harm to this individual if antibiotics are prescribed and the extra time it may take to negotiate a different course of action.

Individuals can operate at different levels at different times (as in the oil spill example) and vary their values depending on the context they are in. Therefore a GP can be all for avoiding antibiotic prescription when in an educational setting or a clinical governance meeting, but still issues penicillin to Mrs Jones when she has a touch of bronchitis.

By contrast, written guidelines tend to be calibrated at the level of authorship. So that a written guidance that is part of the primary care trust's or strategic health authority's systems for managing prescribing will retain these values when it is read in the micro setting. It thus appears dissonant, alien, 'them not us'. The same risk applies to guidance implemented electronically. In fact, one could summarise much of clinical governance as being an attempt to encourage people to understand values of different levels of analysis (or to impose one set of values on another level).

In the previous section we described the way that utterances made by people are enriched by many voices through parody and other mechanisms. The implication is that written guidelines, being calibrated at the level of authorship, may lose this richness, either in the writing or the interpretation. The voice is taken at face value. One of the challenges for computerised decision support is to transmit, or make available to the user, some of these subtleties and nuances.

The triadic consultation (practitioner, patient, computer)

This term was coined by Kay and Purves,[36] though they were not the first to consider the impact of the computer on the sacred space of the consultation in primary care.[36] Kay and Purves' view considers the computer as an agent in the consultation (see also Chapter 3, pp. 40–1). It is based on an appreciation that the electronic medical record is fundamentally different from the paper record in its impact on the doctor–client interaction.

The move towards electronic records has two different effects on the practitioner–client interaction. The first is largely due to the different medium, which allows rapid retrieval of diverse parts of the patient's medical record via a computer screen. Similar information is available in paper records, but it is now available in a different way. The second relates to decision support, guidance and information support that may be embedded in the electronic record (for example in templates), may be triggered by entries into the electronic record (e.g. Prodigy[18]), or may be accessed from the desktop computer (e.g. eBNF or internet resources such as NeLH[37]). This is a new range of information and knowledge that is available to the practitioner as a direct result of using electronic records rather than paper.

The iiCR project[38] has studied the effect of computer use in the consultation, and produced a teaching package that delivers the key messages from the project. It shows that computer use, even for 'old' tasks such as looking up a test result on screen, can be distracting and engaging and carries the potential risk of losing rapport with the patient or not hearing what the patient says. The project also shows how the teaching of simple communication skills can minimise this risk. Using an electronic record also makes it easier to share parts of the record with the patient. Again, it was found in iiCR that there is a set of communication skills that facilitate shared reading from a computer screen.

The huge range of accurate and context-sensitive information and knowledge that can be accessed in real time during the consultation is beginning to change the nature of the practitioner–patient relationship. Whereas the professional used to have knowledge that was not available to the layperson, useful knowledge now resides in the computer system: it is available to both, and the client may observe the professional in the process of learning. This changes relationships: it requires the practitioner to display educational and facilitative skills rather than knowledge and power. It makes it easier to involve the patient in the decision-making process.

Shared decision making

Three models of decision making apply to the expert–client relationship. The GP–patient relationship is but one example of this.

Paternalistic (parental)

Here the possession of knowledge and expertise is taken to confer the right and responsibility for decision making to the expert. Frequently, both parties are happy with this arrangement. 'Doctor knows best'. 'I'm in your hands doctor'. 'You're the doctor: you decide'.

This approach implies a blind faith in the expert's abilities and power. This can be seductive to both parties. Changes in the way that society views the professional mean that acceptance of this paternalistic view is less widespread than it was in the first half of the twentieth century. At the same time, the information revolution is making information available to many people outside the professions.

Informed decision making

This is almost the opposite of the paternalistic approach. Here the expert's role is to present information to the client, so that the client has a full grasp of the issues and consequences of the decision. This explication, which may be quite long, is followed by 'what do you want to do?': potentially handing all responsibility for the decision to the client.

Here, the expert has changed from a dispenser of decisions to a dispenser of information. There are two possible drawbacks to this approach. One is that, consciously or unconsciously, the expert may bias the information presented and so control the decision indirectly. The second is that the client may feel, in turn, bombarded by the information and abandoned by the lack of direction.

Shared decision making

Shared decision making goes beyond the presentation of information to the client. It aims to include the patient in every stage of the decision-making process, so that it becomes truly collaborative. Whereas in the informed decision-making model

Table 7.2 Approaches to shared decision making

	Framing the problem	*Discussing the problem and the decision*	*Making the decision*
Paternalistic	Your blood pressure is too high		You need more tablets to bring it down
Informed	Your blood pressure is too high	1 The risks of high blood pressure are ... 2 Possible ways to reduce your blood pressure are ... 3 Consequences of these treatments are ...	What do you want to do?
Shared	Your blood pressure is 160/90, what do you think about that?	Conversation and negotiation	What shall we do?

the expert is presenting information after he or she has framed the problem, in shared decision making the client's framing of the problem is taken into account.

The differences in approach are summarised in Table 7.2, which is based on a hypothetical consultation with a patient with diabetes, whose glycaemic control is good, but whose blood pressure is 160/90.

There is a lot of evidence emerging from the study of communication skills in the consultation that patient involvement in decision making is associated with both improved adherence to a management plan and also to improved health outcomes. This is particularly true of chronic conditions, but applies more broadly.

In the context of this chapter the shared decision-making approach adds another layer of complexity to the situation. Shared decision making depends on using a conceptual framework that is the exclusive property of neither practitioner nor patient. This requires the emergence of a shared conceptual framework during the course of a consultation or a series of consultations. What is the potential impact of computerised decision support on this?

What decision support systems offer now

As discussed earlier, the chief impact of decision support has been to alter the dynamic of the client–expert encounter. Whereas the expert used to possess exclusive professional knowledge and dispense that to the client, such knowledge is now available to both parties during the consultation and outside of it. This moves the practitioner into facilitative, interpretive, educational and explanatory roles.

Diagnostic decision support

Isabel http://isabel.org.uk is a paediatric decision support system that offers help with differential diagnosis and also treatment algorithms for some conditions. For diagnosis there is an open text field into which the clinician can enter clinical features in free text. The system uses an 'intelligent' combination of technologies to provide a differential diagnosis and links to give more detailed information about each. The technology used is described on www.autonomy.com/Content/Technology/#01 The Isabel site stresses that its contribution is to support rather than replace the clinical judgement of the practitioner on the spot.

Dermis is an aid to dermatological diagnosis. It is provided with some clinical computer systems, for example EMIS. Data entry is by completion of a series of forms that ask for information about size, colour, site and duration of lesions, along with other characteristics. The output of the system is a list of possible diagnoses ranked in probability, and also a link to an image that may confirm the diagnosis offered.

Paper systems abound that offer formal rating of symptoms and contribute to the diagnosis of depression or attention deficit hyperactivity disorder (ADHD) for instance, or the assessment of prostatic symptoms to help determine whether referral or further investigation is needed.

What all these systems do is to take specific features from a multifactorial decision and *weight them*. This is often done in line with entry criteria for clinical trials of treatment, and on the basis of calculation of positive predictive values of the specific items. This gives them an appearance of rationality. But they all rely on the practitioner's interpretation of symptoms and signs. Expert clinicians respond to *overall patterns, rather than specific single items,* and there must be considerable doubt about the accuracy of translation of their impression of a patient into the specific features that are used by these systems.

Prescribing and treatment decision support

Prodigy www.prodigy.nhs.uk is a mixed cognitive and rule-based system founded on guidelines that advise on therapeutic actions such as prescriptions, advice leaflets, referral and investigation. It is triggered by the entry of clinical codes in the electronic record and asks the practitioner to specify a scenario within the overall guidance. For instance, in the guidance for acne vulgaris, there are different scenarios for mild, moderate and severe acne. As well as suggesting therapy groups and specific therapies, Prodigy provides a wealth of information that explains the background and justification of the guidance.

Early in the development of Prodigy some GPs started to show some of this background information to patients, for whom it was not intended. This led to the provision of *shared screens*. These have the potential to be of great use in promoting shared decision making, since they offer to the patient a pick-list of issues relating to a particular condition: this is a third-party conceptual framework. However, when use of shared screens was encouraged in the iiCR project, we found that GP trainers were reluctant to use them.

The Prodigy system relies on the practitioner making the diagnosis and is presented in such a way that only the relevant part of the clinical algorithm is displayed, along with links to further information that may be required. The next release of Prodigy will read other relevant information from the clinical record, so that the guidance offered will be appropriate to the position of the patient on a particular disease trajectory.

Conclusion: how an understanding of complexity theory could improve decision support systems in the future

This chapter started by discussing the three aspects of decision making. This places decision support, tools that encourage rational action in real life, firmly between descriptions of how people really do make decisions and normative views of a rational ideal.

We considered individuals and groups in healthcare as if they are complex systems, and then went on to develop a view of behaviour and decision making through the writings of people whose main disciplines include philosophy, biology, neural science, mathematics, psychology, political science, linguistics and medicine. What came out of this journey is the view that all decisions, whether of individuals alone, of dyads such as the medical consultation, or of larger groups such as practices or health authorities, are emergent and inherently unpredictable. What price decision support and rational decision making now?

However, it is, a mistake to think that by celebrating the emergent we are decrying the rational. Plainly the rational scientific paradigm has achieved a great deal. It is an essential part of our way of making sense of the world. Indeed, according to Stewart and Cohen, it is through our talent for representing the complex world in simple ways that our intelligence and consciousness have evolved. We not only like rationalism, we are stuck with it.

The point, more correctly, is that the rational (as represented by the biomedical sciences) is only one voice in the consultation, and, as we discussed, there are competing voices at play here. The consultation is an in-the-room encounter between two mammals. Large parts of the communication that goes on in this encounter are non-verbal, large parts of the behaviour and decision making are subconscious and automated: it is what we call intuition.

Third, through training, experience and practice, doctors are imbued with the technical-rational model. Actions for which they are prepared and with which they are familiar will be dispatched with similar panache to that shown by the elite sportsman. Again, like the sportsman, these actions will occur automatically without recourse to reflection in action. A tennis player's choice of shot will be influenced by the state of the game, his or her competence (which will depend on skill, practice, rehearsal and training), and his or her confidence and experience. So, while the decision to hit that ball in that way is spontaneous and not under conscious control at the time, it is influenced by many factors that lie outside the theatre of action and can be subject to conscious reflection.

Which leads us to the question: What is the purpose of decision support in healthcare? One purpose is to aid the practitioner with difficult decisions that lie outside or stretch the practitioner's usual expertise. For instance the decision support for the acute abdomen[39] has been used to assist unqualified naval crew in the decision about whether to airlift personnel to hospital. A similar role can be envisaged of supporting nurse practitioners in tasks that have previously been in the medical domain. The assumption here is that there is deliberation in the actions of the practitioner, who is aware that he or she is acting out of the comfort zone. In this environment, the practitioner is acting out the 'hypothetico-deductive reasoning' model. This used to be regarded as the natural modality for clinical reasoning, but in the light of the rest of this chapter, and as is pointed out elsewhere,[40] hypothetico-deductive reasoning is itself a learned schema. In short, the practitioner knows that he or she is under challenge and is stopping to think.

Another purpose of decision support is to encourage consistency across the health service and ensure that best practice is spread. This is one of the aims of clinical governance, and as can be seen in policy documents such as *Information for Health*,[41] it is one of the main justifications for funding electronic records and decision support systems. In this scenario, the intention may be, for instance, to reduce antibiotic prescribing for minor respiratory infections. In this well-rehearsed territory, the practitioner will be more likely to be running on a more intuitive approach to decisions. While the yield for a successful system would be high (in terms of the number of consultations where these common situations arise) it is correspondingly more unlikely that the practitioner will engage with decision support.

The different scenarios outlined in the last two paragraphs lie at opposite ends of the cognitive continuum.[42] At the deliberative end the emergent decision is to seek help. The first task for a decision support system is to present itself as an option and be available for conversation with the rational voice that has already emerged in the practitioner's mind. Priorities here are availability, accessibility, familiarity and ease of use. The latter is particularly important as, by definition, the practitioner is under stress already.

At the low-challenge end of the continuum it is unlikely that the rational voice will be heard at all. In a routine consultation for a common acute condition, such as sore throat, the answer to 'would you like to use decision support?' is likely to be 'no'. While the question may be relevant at the meso and macro levels of analysis, at the micro level of familiar practice it will be seen as an irrelevant distraction. Making technical and rational information easily available is not enough. The decision support system needs to be more involved in the context of practice and in the instant.

One way to achieve this relates to managing chronic conditions, such as hypertension, where simple algorithms become complicated by co-morbidity and multiple prescriptions. The approach used here by the second release of Prodigy is to read information from the clinical record and suggest, and justify, action appropriate to the individual patient at their current point on their disease trajectory.

In common acute conditions, an analogous role would be for the system to track the practitioner's activity over a period of time, and with many patients. What is at issue here are the practitioner's habits, and the role of the system would be to track habitual behaviour and offer reminders. It may often be easier for the practitioner to be presented with this feedback outside of the consultation at a time when there is room for reflection. Educationally, such a system could be very effective, provided that the practitioner was engaged with it. This would require involvement of the practitioner in deciding which conditions were being monitored by the system, and with what criteria. If its introduction were perceived to be political, and the settings made at a different level of analysis, then it would not be used.

In all these potential uses of decision support, the key issue is one of *engagement with the practitioner*. Whether the system is being used in a high-challenge acute situation, in chronic conditions, or in routine acute conditions, the requirement is for conversation between the practitioner and the system. It is not a question of either the individual or the system having the answer, it is for an answer to emerge from the *zone of proximal development* that is represented by the practitioner's interaction with the system. For this to work the practitioner needs to know more about the decision support system and have the ability to customise it. The system needs to know more about what the practitioner is doing. In short, they need to *share context*.

Awareness of this complexity presses one to question current decision support methods, since that support is based on the assumption that decision making is solely a one-way rational process. In fact, the complexity of real-life situations means that first of all, the practitioner, as an agent, is not led by one view (or voice) but by multiple interacting views and levels of analysis. And moreover, the practitioner is not the sole agent within the context of decision making. Consequently, decision-making processes emerge in the specific situation at hand.

References

1   Bazerman M (1988) *Judgement in Management Decision Making* (4e). John Wiley and Sons, Chichester.
2   Edwards W (1971) Social utilities. *Engineering Economist.* Summer symposium series, 6.

3   Elstein A, Shulman L, Sprafka S (1978) *Medical Problem Solving: an analysis of clinical reasoning.* Harvard University Press, London.

4   Schmidt HG, Norman GR, Boshuizen PA (1990) A cognitive perspective on medical expertise. *Theory and Implications Academic Medicine.* **65**: 611–21.

5   Schon DA (1995) *The Reflective Practitioner: how professionals think in action.* Maurice Temple Smith, London, 1983. Reprinted 1995, Arena, Aldershot.

6   Eraut M (1994) *Developing Professional Knowledge and Competence.* Falmer Press, London.

7   Coiera E (1999) Decision support systems. www.coiera.com/ailist/list-main.html#HDR60

8   Kurtz S (1996) The Calgary–Cambridge referenced observation guides: an aid to defining the curriculum and organising the teaching in communication training programmes. *Medical Education.* **30**: 83–9.

9   Searle JR (1969) *Speech Acts: an essay in the philosophy of language.* Cambridge University Press, Cambridge.

10 Bakhtin MM (1986) *Speech Genres and Other Late Essays.* C Emerson, M Holquist (eds). University of Texas Press, Austin.

11 Robinson PJ, Heywood P (2000) What do GPs need to know? The use of knowledge in general practice consultations. *Br J Gen Pract.* **50**: 56–9.

12 Sackett DL, Straus SE, Richardson WS *et al.* (1999) *Evidence-based Medicine: how to practise and teach EBM.* Churchill Livingstone, London.

13 Greenhalgh T, Hurwitz B (1998) *Narrative Based Medicine. Dialogue and Discourse in Clinical Practice.* BMJ Books, London.

14 Muir Gray J (1999) National electronic Library for Health (NeLH) prototype. www.nelh.nhs.uk/strategy.htm

15 Isabel http://isabel.org.uk

16 Dermis www.mentor-update.com/

17 Hospital Anxiety and Depression scale. Accessed from NeLH on www.nelh.nhs.uk/nsf/chd/nsf/pdfs/ch7appndxa-4.pdf

18 Prodigy www.Prodigy.nhs.uk

19 SCHIN (2002) *PRODIGY Evidence Based Clinical Guidelines.* Sowerby Centre for Health Informatics, Newcastle upon Tyne.

20 British Thoracic Society/SIGN (2003) British guideline on the management of asthma. www.brit-thoracic.org.uk/sign/pdf/SIGN63.PDF

21 Stacey RD (2001) *Complex Responsive Processes in Organisations: learning and knowledge creation.* Routledge, London.

22 Stewart I (1997) *Does God Play Dice?* (2e) Penguin, London, p. 57.

23 Kay S, Purves I (1996) Medical records and other stories: a narratological framework. *Methods Inf Med.* **35**: 72–88

24 Dennett DC (1993) *Consciousness Explained.* Penguin Books, London.

25 Dennett DC (1995) *Darwin's Dangerous Idea: evolution and the meanings of life.* Penguin, London.

26 Cohen J, Stewart I (1997) *Figments of Reality: the evolution of the curious mind.* Cambridge University Press, Cambridge.

27 For an overview of this area see: Greenfield S (2000) *Brain Story.* BBC Worldwide, London.

28 For an overview of this area see: Wegner DM (2002) *The Illusion of Conscious Will.* Bradford Books, MIT Press, Cambridge, MA.

29 Libert B (1992) The neural time factor in perception, volition and free will. *Revue de Metaphysique et de Moral.* **97**: 255–72.

30 Edelman G, Tononi G (2000) *A Universe of Consciousness: how matter becomes imagination.* Basic Books, New York.

31 Bartlett FC (1932) *Remembering: an experimental and social study.* Cambridge University Press, Cambridge.

32 Dewey J (1933) *How We Think – a restatement of the relation of reflective thinking to the educative process.* Heath, Boston.

33 Kolb D (1984) *Experiential Learning.* Englewood Cliffs, Prentice Hall, NJ.

34 Blackmore S (1999) *The Meme Machine.* Oxford University Press, Oxford.

35 Wertsch J (1991) *Voices of the Mind: a sociocultural approach to mediated action.* Harvard University Press, Cambridge, MA.

36 Hayes GM (1993) Use of the computer in the consultation. *Update.* **47**(7): 465–8.

37 NeLH www.nelh.nhs.uk/

38 iiCR www.schin.ncl.ac.uk/iiCR

39 De Dombal FT, de Baere H, van Elk PJ *et al.* (1993) Objective medical decision making. Acute abdominal pain. In: JEW Beneken, V Thevenin (eds) *Advances in Biomedical Engineering*, pp. 65–87. IOS Press, Amsterdam.

40 Robinson P, Purves I (2003) Learning support for the consultation: information support and decision support should be placed in an educational framework. *Medical Education.* **37**: 429–33.

41 Department of Health (1998) *Information for Health.* DoH, London, pp. 63, 68.

42 Hamm R (1988) Clinical intuition and clinical analysis: expertise and the cognitive continuum. In: J Dowie, A Elstein (eds) *Professional Judgement: a reader in clinical decision making.* Cambridge University Press, Cambridge.

CHAPTER 8

Improving health outcomes using integrated health informatics and iterative behavioural feedback

Sylvie Robichaud-Ekstrand and Tim Holt

Introduction

The 1990s witnessed two significant developments in the approach of healthcare professionals towards change management. One of these was the widespread introduction of *clinical audit* which, when carried out correctly, involves repeated cycles of data collection and assessment, planned change and reassessment after an interval of time.[1] This mechanism is an example of a recurrently iterated process, in which the most recent state following action implementation becomes the starting conditions for the next cycle. As discussed earlier in this book, this sort of repeated iteration is a fundamental mechanism through which adaptive change occurs in complex systems.

The other development, also very much in keeping with the themes of this book, was the recognition, developed over the past decade by Prochaska and DiClemente,[2,3] that effective interventions require the system to be in a *state of readiness* for change. However obvious the need for lifestyle change may seem to a clinician, attempts to impose it from outside are likely to fall on stony ground if the degree of motivation of the individual is not accounted for.

A third element, which was not available until recently, but is now becoming increasingly important, is the *integration* of information from clinical and other databases, enabling the multiple components of the extended team to interact in ways not previously possible. These databases have also greatly expanded the profiles from which patient groups can be identified, from the rudimentary age/sex registers of the days before computerisation, to the increasingly rich electronic records detailing innumerable factors relevant to change management and risk reduction.

Combined with the ongoing move towards patient involvement and participation, these elements enable us to recognise the complex, context-dependent and changing needs of our patients. This chapter discusses these principles using the example of cardiovascular disease prevention, and describes the Iterative Computer-tailored Feedback System developed in Canada during the late 1990s.

The scale of the problem

Cardiovascular disease (CVD), including heart disease and stroke, is still the major cause of disability, hospital admissions and death, despite evidence that mortality rates are declining. Recent decrease in CVD mortality is partly explained by the decline in population rates of smoking and changes in dietary habits,[4–6] and partly due to improved survival from acute myocardial infarction (AMI).[6] With improved AMI survival, rates of hospitalisation for other types of CVD such as congestive heart failure (CHF) and stroke are on the rise. CVD has therefore become the leading contributor to the global burden of disease with the highest number of disability-adjusted life-years (DALY), a measure that incorporates incidence, prevalence and disability impact.[7,8]

Consider an individual who smokes due to frustration with workplace stress. His lack of coping skills and low motivation prevent him from adopting strategies to quit smoking despite his knowledge that smoking is bad for him and his family circle; no one in his social network supports his frustration or his attempts to quit smoking. His smoking hinders his participation in regular exercise and he becomes more sedentary and more prone to weight gain and hypertension. This further leads to increased LDL-cholesterol and lowered HDL-cholesterol. Clearly, risk factor reduction for this individual is complex. It is multifactorial and would differ from another individual, even one with the same blood pressure and lipid profile but a different affective, behavioural and cognitive profile.

Research has provided much evidence on clinical cardiovascular risk (CV) factors, and on the relationship between health behaviour modification and change in clinical risk factors. Less is known on the extent to which these risk factors *cluster* and lead to disease occurrence and poor quality of life, and the extent to which tailoring risk factor reduction strategies to multifactorial risk factor profiles would decrease the risk of CVD and improve quality of life. Considering the high prevalence of CVD, the diversity in risk profiles, the complexity of managing CV risk and the need to use multi-modal interventions, computers have become the ideal tool to manage the high volume of individuals with CV risk factors at a lesser cost.

The Iterative Computer-tailored Feedback System

The Iterative Computer-tailored Feedback System (ICFS) is an *expert system* whose purpose is to reduce morbidity and mortality outcomes in patients with CVD and/or type 2 diabetes. It is designed to be more widely applicable to the population at large, but has so far been used to target clients currently under the care of a cardiologist or diabetologist. It uses a series of computerised algorithms that manipulate data from medical charts, laboratory data banks and self-administered behavioural questionnaires. It gives feedback on clinical, cognitive and behaviour outcomes by generating tailored reminders and messages in the form of printed letters and pamphlets. A team of interdisciplinary researchers, clinicians and computer science experts in Montreal, Canada, led by Sylvie Robichaud-Ekstrand, and graduate students from three different universities and research centres developed the system. It comprises expert and student nurses, psychologists, cardiologists, endocrinologists, health services and informatics scholars.

The aim of the *computer-tailored reminders* is to relay information between health professionals and patients on modifiable CV risk factors. Since health professionals and patients receive the same information, but in *adapted* formats, awareness and knowledge levels are increased, which provoke discussion during medical visits and augment concordance.

Theoretical models provide the initial structure to select among psychosocial determinants or characteristics that influence behaviour. As theories only represent models of reality, they need to be supported by empirical data, before being translated into intervention message objectives.[9] Two factors to take into account when selecting appropriate determinants are their impact on the desired health outcome(s) and their amenability to produce change in the individuals' affective, cognitive, social, behavioural and/or physiological states. When developing the system, the team decided to utilise Prochaska and DiClemente's Transtheoretical Model[2] (Box 8.1) and Bandura's Self-efficacy Theory[10-12] (Box 8.2), concentrating on stages and processes of change, self-efficacy and concordance, or dissonance between actual and perceived behaviour.

The purpose of the *computer-tailored messages* is to help patients adopt, modify or maintain healthy behaviours. This 'computerised counselling' works at the cognitive and behavioural levels. It provides advice on how to transcend stages of behavioural change by utilising appropriate cognitive processes, identifying coping abilities and augmenting feelings of self-efficacy in tempting situations.

Box 8.1   The Transtheoretical Model[2] – stages and processes of behavioural change

Stages of change reflect patients' readiness to modify behaviour. In the *precontemplation* stage, there is no intention to modify behaviour within at least six months. The client may not realise how their behaviour impacts on their life. *Contemplation* signifies that individuals are becoming aware that their behaviour is problematic, but still feel ambivalence about changing. *Preparation* is the stage that combines intention and behavioural efforts. Individuals therefore project to initiate actions in the next month, as they foresee more advantages than disadvantages in changing. They also feel somewhat to very confident in being able to change their behaviour. *Action* is the time frame where individuals actually modify their behaviours, their relationships, their experiences and their environment. However, habits have not yet been established; hence these individuals are at high risk of relapsing to previous unhealthy behaviours. *Maintenance* includes ways utilised to prevent relapse and to preserve gains acquired at the action stage. When a person does not perceive any more temptation to revert back to an unhealthy behaviour, and he or she feels completely confident, the stage of change is called *termination*. Given that most people do not follow a linear path when modifying behaviour, the model is schematically represented by a cycle, which indicates that many attempts may be necessary before modifying and maintaining a healthy behaviour. Individuals can regress to a previous stage, learn from it and eventually reach the maintenance stage.

Box 8.2   Self-efficacy Theory[10–12]

Self-efficacy, a cognitive determinant of behaviour, represents individuals' confidence to adopt, modify and/or maintain a healthy behaviour when encountering difficult situations. Bandura postulates that individuals derive information that may influence their confidence level from four sources: performance accomplishments, vicarious experience, verbal persuasion, and emotional arousal. *Performance accomplishments* refer to how successful an individual is at performing the task(s) of interest. Effective performance that enhances mastery and is processed cognitively augments self-efficacy. Self-efficacy may be enhanced through *vicarious experience*. Individuals who observe others successfully perform challenging tasks without negative consequences may begin to expect that they could also achieve the same tasks through perseverance. *Verbal persuasion* consists of verbal attempts to convince individuals that they are capable of achieving successful performance. Its effects may depend on whether the individual perceives the persuader to be credible, trustworthy, competent and assured. *Emotional arousal*, such as levels of fear and anxiety, will negatively affect performance and are often interdependent.

How an individual cognitively processes information is important, as successful behaviour and performance may have less of an impact if the person attributes the success to external factors rather than personal skills, if the mastery of a particular task is considered relatively easy, or if the individual's confidence baseline level is low. Weak levels of self-efficacy at onset are more readily diminished by unsuccessful performance. Alternatively, when confidence levels are high, people are little swayed by failure.

It counsels on how to take advantage of available resources and on how to get support from formal and informal social networks. It provides insight on progress, lack of progress on healthy behaviours, or relapse to unhealthy behaviours. Consequently, it places patients at the centre of their care and empowers them to participate in self-care activities intended to increase adherence to medical recommendations and health behaviour modification and maintenance.

The ultimate goal is to improve physical, emotional and social health, and decrease CVD, such as coronary artery disease (CAD), congestive heart failure and stroke.

Computer-tailored reminders identify health professionals responsible for managing specific CV risk factors; and inform and provide feedback to medical practitioners and patients on CV factors requiring tighter control. Cardiovascular risk factors targeted with this system include: lipid profile, glycaemic control, blood pressure, smoking status, weight maintenance, level of physical activities, microalbuminuria, date of last ophthalmologic examination and missed medical visits.

Computer-tailored messages individually assess behaviours and cognitive processes (i.e. self-efficacy, readiness to change, perception of performance, actual behaviour). They provide tailored advice based on these assessments, *relying on patients' identified priorities rather than relative risk*. They integrate information about the cognitive and behavioural patterns that influence health-related decisions and actions of individuals. Behaviours for which tailored advice is provided comprise:

- eating less fat
- participating in regular physical activity
- better stress management
- smoking cessation
- taking medications as prescribed.

Reminders and messages are:

- *personalised*, as patients' and health professionals' names are listed
- *positive*, as desired states are reinforced
- *empathetic*, as the person's feelings, motives and attributed meaning in regard to health behaviours are reiterated
- *informative* on cognitive behavioural states.

Other features of the ICFS comprise:

- the identification of community health and social services (*Centre local de services communautaires* – CLSC) within the vicinity of patients' dwellings which are based on postal, street and municipality codes
- insertion of summaries of clinical guidelines pertaining to specific cardiovascular risk factors requiring tighter control
- presentation of a list of available community, Web and organisation resources
- production of address labels for correspondence
- generation of output data files for statistical analyses.

Why use computer-tailored messages?

It is recognised that GPs seldom have adequate time during an office visit to provide sufficient individual information necessary to tailor counselling on a variety of preventive health behaviours, and then to engage in the counselling. Consequently, patients' active participation may be excluded from the treatment plan. This seems to be even more evident with patients coming from lower socio-economic backgrounds.[13,14] Without adequate counselling and support, cardiac patients will have greater difficulty in making changes towards behaviours that lead to a healthy lifestyle.

Among the modifiable CV risk factors, most medical literature has focused on clinical risk factors such as high blood pressure and elevated lipids and triglycerides. However, as indicated in Table 8.1, affective, behavioural and social factors are also modifiable risk factors, and if modified, can produce positive health outcomes.

Affective factors include signs and symptoms of anxiety, depression, hostility and anger. Behavioural factors include smoking, exercise, diet, stress management, social participation, medication compliance and regular medical visits. Social factors cover extensiveness and structure of the social network, the perception of the availability and quality of support, and frequency of social contacts.[20] Through cognitive processes, knowledge, motivation and coping, this ensemble of modifiable risk factors alters the risk of disease and health-related quality of life. Recent

Table 8.1 Non-modifiable and modifiable cardiovascular risk factors. Adapted from: Devasenapathy and Hachinsk[15]; Dyken and Pokras[16]; Gasecki and Hachinski[17]; Mayo[18,19]

	Non-modifiable	Modifiable
Socio-demographic	Age Male gender Family history Ethnicity	
External factors	Season and climate Socio-economic factors Previous/concomitant life events	Geographic location Political climate Community/environment
Affective factors		Depression/anxiety Hostility/anger Moods
Social factors		Social support Social capital

Health behaviour		Cigarette smoking
		Sedentary lifestyle
		Obesity/overweight
		Diet (high fat/high sugar/
		  low fibre)
		Non-adherence to
		  pharmacologic treatments
		
		Alcohol abuse
		Oral contraceptives
		Illicit drug abuse

Clinical factors directly related to CVD	Previous stroke
	
	Previous myocardial
	  infarction
		Hypertension
		Dyslipidaemia
		Hypercholesterolaemia,
		Hypertriglyceridaemia
		Low HDL-cholesterol
		Diabetes Glucose intolerance,
		      Insulin resistance,
		      Hyperinsulinaemia
		Elevated fibrinogen
		Elevated haematocrit
		Homocystine
		
		Ischaemic heart disease
		Valvular heart disease
		Left ventricular hypertrophy
		Peripheral vascular disease
		Atrial fibrillation
		Transient ischaemic attack
		Carotid stenosis/bruits

Other clinical factors		Migraine; Sickle cell disease; Lupus anticoagulant; Anticardiolipin antibodies; Hyperuricaemia; Infection/febrile illness

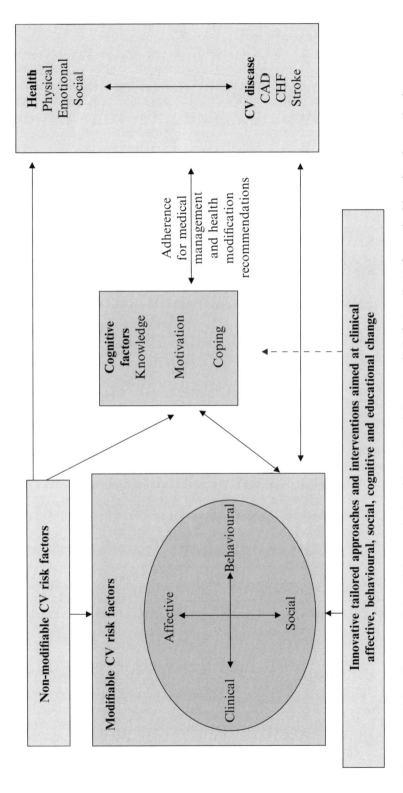

Figure 8.1   Schematic representation of the complexity of interactions between multiple factors that influence health and cardiovascular disease.

evidence suggests that risk factors for CAD and stroke are interactive in their effects, underlining the importance of tackling all major risk factors rather than concentrating on one single factor.

Each CV risk factor carries independently or in combination with others, a degree of morbidity and a negative impact on quality of life affected by health. Factors are also influenced by *external* forces such as geographic location, season and climate, socio-economic factors, political climate, community/environment and previous or concomitant life events.

The hypothesised mechanism whereby the use of the ICFS might impact on the occurrence of CVD is through improved adherence to recommendations for medical management and health modification recommendations (Figure 8.1). Support for this hypothesis comes from evidence that highly motivated persons can make drastic lifestyle changes that lead to improved cardiovascular health,[21] even without medications.[22]

Why develop computer-tailored information?

There are good reasons to believe that computer-tailored information will have much greater impact on behavioural change in individuals than more generalised information. Tailored material is more likely to be read completely, discussed with others, and found to contain more relevant, interesting and new information when compared to general or targeted materials.[23–27]

Six systematic reviews on *Computer-based Decision Support Systems* (CDSS), which include 68 randomised clinical trials between 1974 and 1998, present enough data to confirm that the use of CDSS can affect clinicians' and patients' behaviour in regard to managing cardiovascular risk.[28–34] Over the years, expert systems have evolved and started to incorporate various psychosocial determinants of behavioural change, based on theoretical and conceptual frameworks.

Campbell *et al.*[35] tested the effect of receiving tailored nutrition messages to decrease fat intake and increase fruit and vegetable intake in primary care settings. Total fat intake decreased by 23% in the tailored group; and by 9% and 3% in the non-tailored (1990 Dietary Guidelines for Americans) and control groups respectively. Later, Campbell and colleagues[36] reported that a computer-tailored self-help health promotion programme may be an effective educational intervention for lower income and minority groups. Brug *et al.*[37] reported that computer-tailored feedback had a greater impact on fat reduction and augmentation of fruit and vegetable intake than did general information. Iterative computer-tailored feedback produced an even greater impact.

Cardinal and Sachs[38] increased physical activity using the stages of change model and mail-delivered exercise programmes. Even though non-computerised, these researchers were the first ones to tailor messages for exercising according to stage of change, in conjunction with predicted cardiorespiratory fitness and percentage body fat. Results also indicated that more subjects progressed through the stages of change (28.7%) than relapsed (9.3%).

Most studies using computer-tailored feedback systems have been performed in the area of smoking cessation, and have demonstrated significant effects. Prochaska *et al.*[39] reported that at 6, 12 and 18 months, the stage-matched manuals group had double the smoking cessation rate of the self-help manuals. Over 18 months, the most effective group was the combination of interactive expert-system computer reports, plus individualised manuals group, demonstrating the highest smoking cessation rate and prolonged abstinence rates. Strecher *et al.*[40] evaluated the effects of computer-tailored smoking cessation messages in family practice settings. Results from their two studies indicated that tailored messages in the format of letters among moderate to light smokers increased smoking cessation (30.7% and 19% respectively) compared to the control group (7.1% and 7.3% respectively). The messages were tailored according to cigarette consumption, interest in quitting smoking, perceived benefits and barriers to quitting, and other factors relevant to smoking cessation.

These previous studies on computer-tailored feedback systems confirm their effectiveness to modify certain individual behaviours in specific areas over other interventions. New data collection modalities that will improve efficiencies in the process of computerised tailoring include the World Wide Web, interactive multimedia through CD-ROM, kiosk, interactive voice response and personal digital assistants.[41] However, the emphasis will always remain on the *quality of tailoring*, which only expert systems can do, based on determinants identified from multiple theoretical models and empirical data.

A matter of impact

Impact is the product of efficacy and participation rate.[42,43] Efficacy refers to the power of the intervention enabling patients to progress to higher levels of stage of change that lead to the adoption and maintenance of a healthy behaviour. Participation rate is determined by the number of patients within a specific population who participate in the intervention. Using smoking cessation as an example (Table 8.2), previous studies[36,37] have shown that expert systems produce both high effectiveness and participation rates, resulting in an 18% impact rate for smoking cessation. Smoking cessation clinics and pharmacological agents are known to be successful in producing high smoking cessation rates (30%). However, their utilisation rate is low (1% to 3%). Consequently, their impact effect (0.03% to 0.09%) has been found to be lower than that of simple medical advice (0.3%). Therefore, it seems logical that expert systems have the potential to be more cost-effective by tailoring the information and having the capability to reach more

Table 8.2   Impact of various smoking cessation interventions (from Velicer WF *et al.*)[42]

Intervention	Effectiveness rate (%)	Participation rate (%)	Impact rate (%)
Expert system	22–26	75	18
Smoking cessation clinics	30	1	0.03
Pharmacological treatment	30	3	0.09
Self-help manual	15	5	0.75
Medical advice	10	30	0.3
Community intervention	1	80	0.08

individuals, at lower costs. The financial burden on the healthcare system could therefore be substantially reduced.

Generating tailored messages and reminders

Message objectives are formulated to attain desired cognitive and behavioural outcomes. First of all, specific information related to targeted behaviours or cognitions is collected on individuals by administering a questionnaire, performing a telephone survey or having participants enter their responses directly into the computer. Second, algorithms are developed to incorporate these data and generate reminders or messages in a predetermined format. To date, computerised expert systems have generated them in the form of letters, computer printouts, newsletters, magazines, personal diaries, greeting cards, correspondence courses, bible statements and electronic messages on computer screen.

The functions of the ICFS include:

- the importation of raw data from patient medical charts and questionnaires into tables within the expert system database
- the running of algorithms utilising raw data to create intermediate variables and/or feedback variables (selection of tailored messages from a series of algorithms)
- the computer diagnosis of medical conditions according to clinical guidelines (i.e. hypertension, hyperlipidaemia, diabetes)
- the retrieving of messages from libraries
- the creation of tailored printed information in the form of pamphlets and letters incorporating reminders and messages, in Word page format
- the display and printing of personalised and standard letters, envelopes, labels used for correspondence
- the tracking and reporting of the number of times a specific exit within a given algorithm is selected, thus accounting for the iterative component of the expert system
- the generation of data files, ready for manipulation with statistical programs (as each table within the database stores a series of distinct variables for all subjects, an additional program merges these files together)
- the creation of a temporary table of new medications, not yet incorporated into the expert system.

Feedback can be *normative* (when messages compare individuals states to those of comparable others); *iterative* (when additional data collected at subsequent times is used in the feedback system); *personalised* (if the person's name is listed); *positive* (when desired states are reinforced); *empathetic* (when understanding of the person's feelings is reiterated); or it can offer information on cognitive behavioral states (e.g. self-efficacy).[44]

Messages can also invite telephone or computer interactive counselling that mimics face-to-face counselling with a health professional. Thus there exist many varieties of tailoring.[45] Advances in computer technology make it easier and more cost-effective to produce large quantities of tailored information in a limited time,[46] or provide immediate feedback. The number of output permutations increases

Table 8.3 Examples of messages according to strategies for various experiential cognitive processes of change

Process of change	Example of suggested strategy	Examples of messages
Consciousness raising	Provide indication and written materials about the risks of not adopting the healthy behaviour	'Did you know that cigarettes are your heart's number one enemy? Smoking is the most important risk factor for developing fatty deposits in your body's arteries (atherosclerosis); it increases your levels of bad cholesterol (LDL), while decreasing the level of good cholesterol (HDL)'
Dramatic relief	Allow the person to express how he feels about being a smoker or quitting smoking	'How do I feel as a smoker?' 'How do I feel about quitting smoking?'
Environmental evaluation	Provide evidence for increased illness risks if not adopting the healthy behaviour	'We understand the difficulties people face in quitting, given the physical and psychological addiction many people have. However, we encourage you to recognise the terrible effects cigarettes have on your health, and to take the time to consider your smoking status'
Self-re-evaluation	Use imagery to increase emotional awareness	'Imagine how you would feel if you were exercising more regularly; the wellbeing, both physical and psychological, that you would feel. This exercise might help you to better visualise the benefits of this healthy habit'
Social liberation	Point out people who included this healthy behaviour in their lives	'You could speak with someone in your circle of friends who exercises regularly and who might be able to provide support and encouragement. Ask how he or she integrates exercise into his or her daily routine without missing out on his or her social life, for example'
Experiential	Believing in one's ability to change	'The days when you feel most self-confident and motivated are the times to initiate even bigger changes. You would feel even more self-confidence when you realise that you can change such behaviours'

exponentially with the number of individual characteristics to be included into the tailored iterative feedback system.[47,48] This further confirms the need to computerise content material, when tailoring is desired. Tables 8.3 and 8.4 give examples of the tailoring of messages according to alternative strategies selected, and the client's level of self-efficacy.

How does the ICFS fit into the bigger scheme of things?

Although the ICFS is electronic, it is currently being filled in by a research nurse using data abstracted from medical charts and laboratory databases. Once the impact of the ICFS is known, our involvement with the the Integrated Health Research Network (**I**nfostructure de **R**echerche **I**ntégrée en **S**anté au Québec) (Project IRIS-Quebec) and the Cyber-Santé project will permit this tool to become completely electronic by having access to population-level healthcare databases.

The Integrated Health Research Network consists of a consortium of four University Hospital Centres affiliated to the four Quebec Faculties of Medicine with their Research Institutes on one hand, and three Regional Councils for Health and Social Services with their respective Technocentres on the other hand (Quebec Province, Canada) (see Figure 8.2). This network is presently creating a platform to develop a comprehensive and long-term approach to integrated clinical informatics. Its infrastructure will dramatically enhance the capacity to conduct innovative clinical and population health interventions and research, and promptly introduce evidence-based data into practice. Project IRIS-Quebec is under the direction of Dr Robyn Tamblyn at the Department of Medicine, Epidemiology and Biostatistics of McGill University, Montreal.

At the moment, these databases incorporate the RAMQ (Régie de l'Assurance Maladie du Québec) Medical Insurance Warehouse (pharmaceutical services, medical services, beneficiary database, physician database). In the next three to five years, the Integrated Health Research Network will link to electronic patient records, hospitalisation database, trauma registry, birth registry, cancer registry, vital statistics, air pollution, weather and water databases. With appropriate safeguards concerning confidentiality, this integration will provide easily accessible information routinely for clinical and research purposes.

Summary

The challenge of health promotion for the twenty-first century lies in the enormous numbers of clients requiring support, the plurality of risk factors and personal characteristics relevant to disease outcomes, the wide variation in clients' state of motivation and the increasing tendency towards specialisation in medicine, which threaten to reduce the healthcare system to a number of potentially isolated component parts. A coordinated approach needs to recognise not only the whole range of elements in the system, but also the interactions between them. This applies whether we are considering risk factors in an individual, which often appear to *cluster* and conspire to resist change; or the components of the healthcare

Table 8.4 Examples of messages when levels of self-efficacy are low or medium, when encountering selected difficult situations

Low or medium self-efficacy for stress management when dealing with deadlines	'A major source of stress for many of us is a lack of time. If only there were more hours in the day ... Identify your priorities for the day; before your day begins make a list of your tasks for the day. First, cross out any that are not essential. Next, prioritise those that remain. Remember that your decisions do affect others, for example, your family and friends. Tick off tasks as they are completed; this brings satisfaction and it lowers your stress level. Anything left on the list at the end of the day goes on the next day's list. Focus on one task at a time; anything that deserves to be done, deserves to be done well'
Low or medium self-efficacy for exercising and making excuses	'It seems that you frequently find reasons not to exercise. Perhaps you should write out a contract with yourself, with a reward when the contract is completed. For example, sign a paper promising yourself that you will exercise for 30 minutes, three times a week for a month, with no excuses. Then, reward yourself with a trip to the movies or some other activity you enjoy. In this way you develop the habit of exercising and you will find it easier to continue exercising even after your contract expires. You might also feel guiltier breaking deals that you have made with yourself, knowing that you will not have earned the reward. Be honest with yourself, and good luck!'
Low or medium self-efficacy for smoking cessation during social situations	'It seems you are more inclined to smoke at parties or when with friends or family who also smoke. First of all, when you quit smoking, let everyone around you know. The smokers in your entourage will perhaps be less likely to smoke around you, or to invite you out for a cigarette on a coffee break. You will see how encouraging it is to feel the admiration of people who have gone through the same situation, as most smokers have tried to quit at least once, and know how tough it can be to resist the urge. On the other hand, if you feel that there are some in your group who are hindering your efforts, try to avoid them in your moments of temptation. Believe us; these people are not helping you out. Also, without cutting out your social life entirely, try to stay in on the days when you feel most vulnerable. You will feel less pressure to cheat and to relapse. Finally, try to change your habits that were related to smoking. For example, if you used to have a coffee and a cigarette with a friend, order a juice instead, or propose a walk. This way you will kill two birds with one stone; cutting out cigarettes and exercising regularly. Keep it up! Tempting situations will fade away; believe us!'

These might apply to the individual mentioned earlier in the chapter who smokes due to frustration with workplace stress, leading to infrequent exercise, and lacks support from his social network to quit.

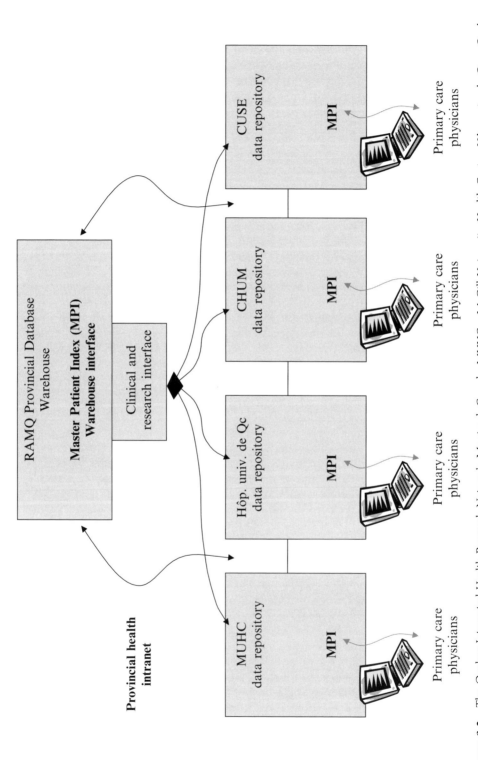

Figure 8.2 The Quebec Integrated Health Research Network, Montreal, Canada. MUHC = McGill University Health Centre; Hôp. univ. de Qc = Quebec University Hospitals; CHUM = Centre Hospitalier de l'Université de Montréal (University of Montreal Health Centre); CUSE = Centre Universitaire de Santé de l'Estrie (Estrie University Health Centre).

team, whose efforts in isolation can be enormously amplified in terms of impact when linked together effectively. In practice, such linkage requires the integration of electronic data from different sources, the generation of tailored advice and information through algorithms that are capable themselves of modification in the light of new research evidence, and an iterative process of feedback that continually reinforces positive outcomes to the central element in the system – the client. The Iterative Computer-tailored Feedback System – described in this chapter may provide a new and effective model, widely applicable in other areas of healthcare, through which these goals can be achieved.

References

1   Marinker M (ed.) (1995) *Medical Audit and General Practice*. BMJ Publishing Group, London.
2   Prochaska JO, DiClemente CC (1992) Stages of change in the modification of problem behaviours. In: M Hersen, RM Eilser, PM Miller (eds) *Progress in Behaviour Modification*, pp. 184–214. Sycamore Press, Sycamore, IL.
3   Prochaska JO, DiClemente CC, Norcross JC (1992) In search of how people change. Application to addictive behaviours. *American Psychologist*. **47**: 1102–14.
4   Beaglehole R (1990) International trends in coronary heart disease mortality, morbidity, and risk factors. *Epidemiol Rev*. **12**: 1–15.
5   Appels A, Jenkins CD, Rosenman RH (1982) Coronary-prone behavior in the Netherlands: a cross cultural validation study. *J Behav Med*. **5**(1): 83–90.
6   Heart and Stroke Foundation of Canada (1999) *The Changing Face of Heart Disease and Stroke in Canada 2000*. Heart and Stroke Foundation of Canada, Ottawa.
7   Murray CJ, Lopez AD (1997) Alternative projections of mortality and disability by cause 1990–2020: Global Burden of Disease Study. *Lancet*. **349**: 1498–504.
8   Murray CJ, Lopez AD (1997) Global mortality, disability, and the contribution of risk factors: Global Burden of Disease Study. *Lancet*. **349**: 1436–42.
9   Dijkstra A, De Vries H (1999) The development of computer-generated tailored interventions. *Patient Education and Counseling*. **36**: 193–203.
10 Bandura A (1977) *Social Learning Theory*. Prentice-Hall, Englewood Cliffs, NJ.
11 Bandura A (1977) Self-efficacy: toward a unifying theory of behavioral change. *Psychol Rev*. **84**(2): 191–215.
12 Bandura A (1997) The anatomy of stages of change. *American Journal of Health Promotion*. **12**(1): 8–10.
13 Paquet G (1994) Facteurs sociaux de la santé, de la maladie et de la mort. In: F Dumont, S Langlois, Y Martin (eds) *Traité des problèmes sociaux*, pp. 223–44. IQRC, Québec.
14 Waller D, Agass M, Mant D *et al*. (1990) Health checks in general practice: another example of inverse care? *BMJ*. **300**: 1115–18.
15 Devasenapathy A, Hachinski V (1998) In: R Teasell (ed.) *Stroke Rehabilitation*, Vol. 12, pp. 367–85. Hanley & Belfus, Inc., Philadelphia, PA.

16 Dyken ML, Pokras R (1984) The performance of endarterectomy for disease of the extracranial arteries of the head. *Stroke.* **15**(6): 948–50.

17 Gasecki A, Hachinski V (1993) In: R Teasell (ed.) *Long-term Consequences of Stroke,* Vol. 7, pp. 43–54. Hanley & Belfus, Inc., Philadephia, PA.

18 Mayo N (1993) In: R Teasell (ed.) *Long-term Consequences of Stroke,* Vol. 7, pp. 1–25. Hanley & Belfus, Inc., Philadephia, PA.

19 Mayo N (1998) In: R Teasell (ed.) *Stroke Rehabilitation,* Vol. 12, pp. 355–66. Hanley & Belfus, Inc., Philadelphia, PA.

20 Barrera M Jr, Ainlay SL (1983) The structure of social support: a conceptual and empirical analysis. *J Community Psychol.* **11**(2): 133–43.

21 Ornish D, Scherwitz LW, Billings JH *et al.* (1998) Intensive lifestyle changes for reversal of coronary heart disease. *JAMA.* **280**(23): 2001–7.

22 Sebregts EH, Falger PR, Bar FW (2000) Risk factor modification through non-pharmacological interventions in patients with coronary heart disease. *J Psychosom Res.* **48**(4–5): 425–41.

23 Strecher VJ, Kreuter M, Den Boer DJ *et al.* (1994) The effects of computer-tailored smoking cessation messages in family practice settings. *J Fam Pract.* **39**(3): 262–70.

24 Skinner CS, Strecher VJ, Hospers H (1994) Physicians' recommendations for mammography: Do tailored messages make a difference? *American Journal of Public Health.* **84**(1): 43–9.

25 Curry SJ, McBride C, Grothaus LC *et al.* (1995) A randomized trial of self-help materials, personalized feedback, and telephone counselling with nonvolunteer smokers. *J Consult Clin Psychol.* **63**(6): 1005–14.

26 Campbell MK, DeVellis BM, Strecher VJ *et al.* (1994) Improving dietary behavior: the effectiveness of tailored messages in primary care settings. *Am J Public Health.* **84**(5): 783–7.

27 Brug J, Steenhuis I, van Assema P *et al.* (1996) The impact of a computer-tailored nutrition intervention. *Preventive Medicine.* **25**: 236–43.

28 Austin SM, Balas EA, Mitchell JA *et al.* (1994) Effect of physician reminders on preventive care: meta-analysis of randomized clinical trials. *Proc Annu Symp Comput Appl Med Care,* pp. 121–4.

29 Balas EA, Austin SM, Mitchell JA *et al.* (1996) The clinical value of computerized information services: a review of 98 randomized clinical trials. *Archives of Family Medicine.* **5**: 271–8.

30 Johnston ME, Langton KB, Haynes RB *et al.* (1994) Effects of computer-based clinical decision support systems on clinician performance and patient outcome: a critical appraisal of research. *Annals of Internal Medicine.* **120**(2): 135–42.

31 Haynes R, Wang E, Da Mota Gomes M (1987) A critical review of interventions to improve compliance with prescribed medications. *Patient Education and Counseling.* **10**: 155–66.

32 Hunt DL, Haynes RB, Hanna SE *et al.* (1998) Effects of computer-based clinical decision support systems on physician performance and patient outcomes. *JAMA.* **280**(15): 1339–46.

33 Shea S, Sideli RV, DuMouchel W *et al.* (1995) Computer-generated informational messages directed to physicians: effect on length of hospital stay. *Journal Am Med Inform Assoc.* **2**: 58–64.

34   Shea S, DuMouchel W, Bahamonde L (1996) A meta-analysis of 16 random-ized controlled trials to evaluate computer-based reminder systems for preventive care in the ambulatory setting. *J Am Med Inform Assoc.* **3**: 399–409.

35   Campbell MK, DeVellis BM, Strecher VJ *et al.* (1994) Improving dietary behavior: the effectiveness of tailored messages in primary care settings. *Am J Public Health.* **84**(5): 783–7.

36   Campbell MK, Honess-Morreale L, Farrell D *et al.* (1999) A tailored multi-media nutrition education pilot program for low-income women receiving food assistance. *Health Education Research.* **14**(2): 257–67.

37   Brug J, Glanz K, van Assema P *et al.* (1998) The impact of computer-tailored feedback and iterative feedback on fat, fruit, and vegetable intake. *Health Education & Behavior.* **25**(4): 517–31.

38   Cardinal BJ, Sachs MC (1993) Increasing physical activity using the stages of change model and mail-delivered exercise program. *Research Quarterly for Exercise and Sport.* **65**: A45.

39   Prochaska JO, DiClemente CC, Velicer WF *et al.* (1993) Standardized, individualized, interactive, and personalized self-help programs for smoking cessation. *Health Psychology.* **12**(5): 399–405.

40   Strecher VJ, Kreuter M, Den Boer DJ *et al.* (1994) The effects of computer-tailored smoking cessation messages in family practice settings. *J Fam Pract.* **39**(3): 262–70.

41   Strecher VJ (1999) Computer-tailored smoking cessation materials: a review and discussion. *Patient Education and Counseling.* **36**(2): 107–17.

42   Velicer WF, Prochaska JO, Fava JL *et al.* (1999) Interactive versus non-interactive interventions and dose-response relationships for stage-matched smoking cessation programs in a managed care setting. *Health Psychology.* **18**(1): 21–8.

43   Velicer WF, Prochaska JO (1999) An expert system intervention for smoking cessation. *Patient Education and Counseling.* **36**: 119–29.

44   Rossi RA, Every NR (1997) A computerized intervention to decrease the use of calcium channel blockers in hypertension. *Journal of General Internal Medicine.* **12**: 672–8.

45   McDonald CJ (1976) Use of a computer to detect and respond to clinical events: its effect on clinician behavior. *Annals of Internal Medicine.* **84**: 162–7.

46   Mazzuca SA, Vinicor F, Einterz WM *et al.* (1990) Effects of the clinical environment on physicians' response to postgraduate medical education. *Am Educ Res J.* **27**: 473–88.

47   Lobach DF, Hammond WE (1994) Development and evaluation of a computer-assisted management protocol (CAMP): improved compliance with care guidelines for diabetes mellitus. *Proc Annu Symp Comput Appl Med Care,* pp. 787–91.

48   Nilasena DS, Lincoln MJ (1995) A computer-generated reminder system improves physician compliance with diabetes preventive care guidelines. *Proc Annu Symp Comput Appl Med Care,* pp. 640–5.

CHAPTER 9

Complex pattern recognition in health data

Lucila Ohno-Machado and Tim Holt

Pattern recognition is important in numerous scenarios in healthcare. It is involved in interpreting diagnostic test results, in recognising patterns of symptoms and signs, in predicting outcomes for seriously ill patients and in searching the electronic information generated in healthcare databases during clinical care. Complex approaches to pattern recognition in these situations may go a long way towards making healthcare both more cost-effective and more adequately tailored to individual patients. The question to be addressed here is: How can complex pattern recognition techniques improve on simpler alternatives to maximise the usefulness of the information we hold?

While the consultation is likely to remain the focal point of clinical care, much of what we do involves the handling of electronically recorded information to target effective clinical interventions, screening or diagnostic tests at the individuals most likely to benefit. The data we hold constitute a dynamic, evolving repository of information, a *'living epidemiology'*.[1] Recognising patterns in an evolving dataset is therefore an essential tool in the delivery of clinical care.

Examples of increasing search protocol complexity

At its most basic level, a simple electronic search on a practice population might involve a single subgroup − for instance a search for those patients with diabetes (remembering that the patients identified by searching on the Diabetes code are not the same as the population subgroup with diabetes; Figure 9.1).

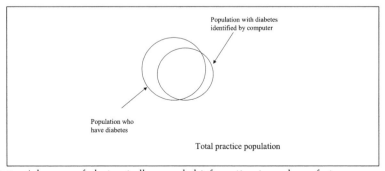

Figure 9.1   Adequacy of electronically recorded information is rarely perfect.

Data quality assurance involves an ongoing effort to make the two circles in Figure 9.1 coincide as closely as possible, i.e. making sure that all patients with diabetes are recorded as such and that no others are. The circles are changing in size all the time, as patients moving into the diabetes group replace those who leave it at variable rates. Because diabetes is usually a 'one-way ticket' diagnosis, the patients only leave the group by dying, but for a different condition (such as colonic cancer or asthma) they might leave it through being cured or through the disorder resolving.

Searching on an assigned Diabetes code identifies an *asymmetry* in the population – distinguishing those with and without diabetes. This basic type of asymmetry is the simplest form of pattern recognition in the data. In the case of diabetes, an individual case can usually be placed either inside or outside of this set. There are borderline states (impaired glucose tolerance and impaired fasting glycaemia) that make the boundary less distinct, but the boundary is defined only in terms of blood glucose levels. In structural terms, we therefore have an asymmetry in the data defined using a single criterion, with a slightly fuzzy boundary. In dynamical terms, we have a subset of the practice's patients whose members enter through being diagnosed and leave through dying.

Few classes in medicine can be defined on the basis of a single criterion. The majority require that a number of factors be taken into account. In terms of search strategies, this then involves the use of more than one search parameter, combined using the Boolean functions AND and OR, or combinations of them.

Venn diagrams such as that in Figure 9.1 are useful for representing different categories that potentially overlap. In order to identify classes using continuous variables, let us imagine plotting a space of possible values for each variable. The dimension of this space is determined by the number of variables involved. Figure 9.2 shows a two-dimensional space, with a single linear 'decision boundary' separating most cases (marked as x) from most non-cases (marked as o).

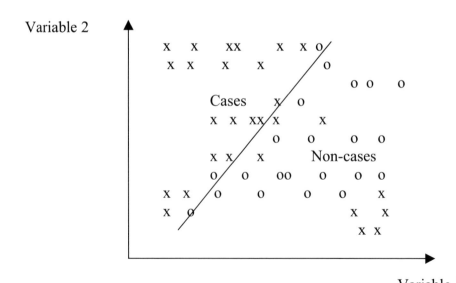

Figure 9.2 A single straight line defines a boundary between most cases and most non-cases, but there is some overlap.

As we will discuss below, linear classification models generally separate cases from non-cases according to single decision boundaries that have a dimension of $n - 1$, where n is the dimension of the space, i.e. the number of variables involved. Such problems are said to be linearly separable, and can be handled well by models such as logistic regression. These include the majority of classification problems we come across. The questions to be addressed in this chapter are:

- how can more complex models deal with classes that are not linearly separable?
- can we usefully identify more complex structures and construct more flexible decision boundaries?

Linear inseparability

Linearly inseparable classes require more complex decision boundaries than their linearly separable counterparts. For example, it may be that a single decision boundary of dimension n or higher needs to be used to separate the cases accurately. Alternatively, there may be a region of the space that is isolated from the region where most cases exist, and therefore requires more than one line or plane to define it. See Figure 9.3 for an illustration of high-dimensional boundaries.

Again, such a classification is only useful if the high-dimensional boundary is a consistent one that separates the classes more reliably than a linear surface. In a large proportion of medical classification problems, linear models suffice. In fact, there are advantages to using linear models in cases where they classify cases well, as there is a risk of 'over-fitting' if more complex structure is assumed where in fact the overlap effect is due to random noise.[2]

Difficult classification problems are commonplace in medicine, but are they *complex*, in the sense implied above? Let us look at two possible examples: the

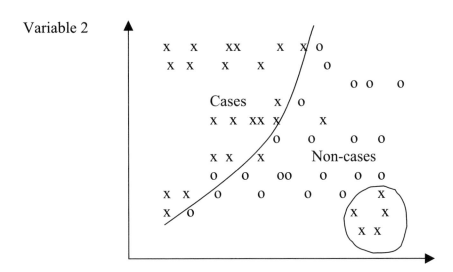

Figure 9.3   A high-dimensional decision boundary improves the specificity and sensitivity of case detection. In addition, a region isolated from the area where most cases are found has been identified.

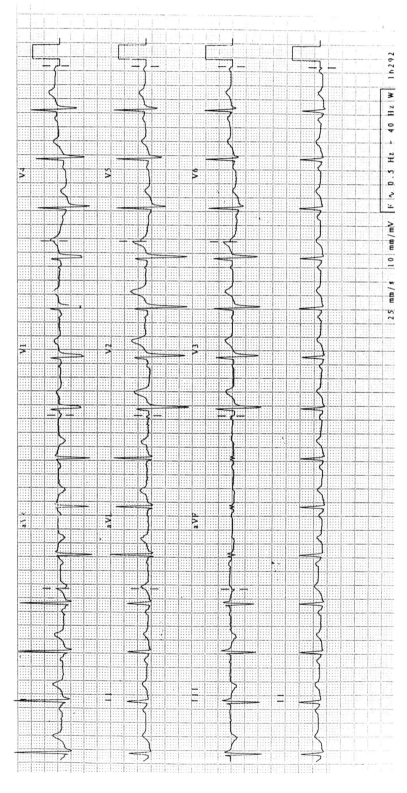

Figure 9.4 ECG from a patient whose LVH was diagnosed purely on the aVL criterion.

electrocardiographic (ECG) diagnosis of left ventricular hypertrophy (LVH), and the identification of patients at risk of heart disease.

Recognising left ventricular hypertrophy by electrocardiography

A simple technique frequently used by clinicians in primary care for the ECG diagnosis of left ventricular hypertrophy (LVH) has been to add the voltage of the tallest R wave in chest leads V5 or V6 to the voltage of the S wave in V1. (In the following discussion, millimetres of amplitude on the ECG paper will be used as units of voltage.) If the sum of these two measurements is greater than 35 mm then the ECG diagnosis of LVH can be made (valid for patients greater than 25 years of age).[3]

However, if the height of the R wave in lead aVL is greater than 13 mm this also suggests LVH, regardless of chest lead criteria values. So there is more than one possible criterion on which to base the diagnosis of LVH. Figure 9.4 gives an example of an ECG from a patient whose LVH was diagnosed purely on the aVL criterion and subsequently confirmed by echocardiography. A simple algorithm for identifying LVH on ECGs might therefore require a single input parameter to be greater than a threshold value:

Criterion 1: (Voltage of R wave in aVL > 13 mm) indicates LVH

All ECGs could be classified using this criterion, but many LVH cases would be missed. The criterion on its own has relatively high specificity but low sensitivity.

Alternatively, the diagnosis might involve a *summation* of two inputs:

Criterion 2: (S wave voltage in V1)
$\left.\begin{array}{c}\text{\textbf{plus}}\\ \text{\textbf{(R wave voltage in V5 or V6)}}\end{array}\right\}$ **> 35 mm indicates LVH**

The possible combinations of inputs fulfilling this second criterion are numerous, as shown in Table 9.1.

So we can now recognise LVH cases according to the fulfilment of *either of two* different criteria, Criterion 1 *or* Criterion 2, increasing the sensitivity of our case detection.

Table 9.1   Combinations of inputs fulfilling criterion 2

V1 voltage	V5 or V6 voltage
10	>25
11	>24
12	>23
13	>22
14	>21
15	>20 . . . etc

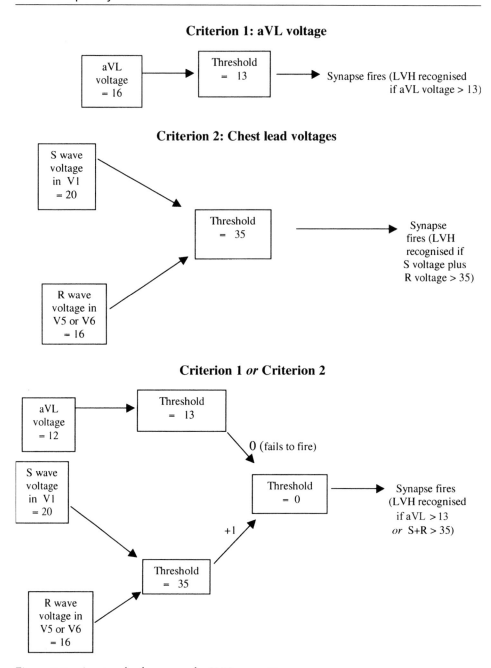

Figure 9.5 A network of synapses for LVH recognition.

Now imagine a more borderline case, where the R wave in aVL was 12 mm, falling short of the diagnostic threshold, and the summation of the chest lead voltages was only 35 mm. Neither criterion would allow the diagnosis on its own, but the *combination* might be highly suggestive. So as well as a simple threshold diagnosis based on a single input (Criterion 1) or a simple summation of inputs (Criterion 2),

Criterion 3: The firing threshold of the initial synapses is reduced, but *both* must fire to recognise LVH

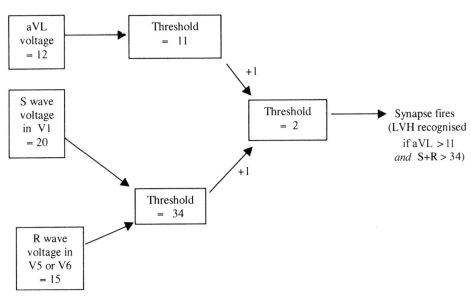

Figure 9.6 The firing threshold of the initial synapses is reduced, but *both* must fire to recognise LVH.

we might allow the 'AND' operator to recognise cases by cross-combining different categories:

> **Criterion 3: Criterion 1 (minus 2 mm)**
> **AND Criterion 2 (minus 1 mm) also suggests LVH**

In this way, a still more sensitive technique for recognising possible LVH has been created which will help to distinguish borderline cases, still based on a very simple algorithm. This pattern recognition technique is illustrated in Figures 9.5 and 9.6 as a network of synapses.

Decision boundaries in the multivariate space of ECG voltages

As the number of variables in the system increases, we are dealing with a classification problem of increasing dimensions. Let us now imagine each variable as an axis so that we can identify areas or regions of the space that correspond to LVH status (Figures 9.7 and 9.8).

Imagine that we now add an additional variable, the voltage of the R wave in the aVR lead, which suggests LVH if greater than 20 mm (Figure 9.10). We can now see that the LVH region is in a three-dimensional space and corresponds to the volume outside the box in Figure 9.10. Adding more relevant variables will progressively increase the dimension of the space and of the boundary, distinguishing cases from

No LVH   LVH

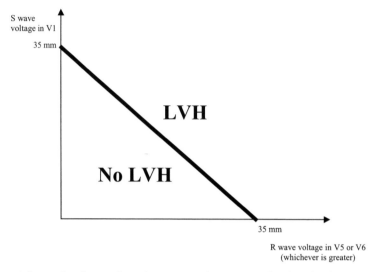

13 mm

aVL R wave voltage

Figure 9.7 A linear classification boundary in one dimension. A single axis ($n = 1$) with a point at 13 mm separating LVH cases from non-cases according to the aVL criterion. There is just one dimension (variable) used, and a single point defines the boundary.

S wave
voltage in V1

35 mm

LVH

No LVH

35 mm

R wave voltage in V5 or V6
(whichever is greater)

Figure 9.8 A linear classification boundary in two dimensions. The chest lead criteria separate LVH cases from non-cases using a single line. The space is two-dimensional, the decision boundary one-dimensional. This decision line could be easily represented using a simple algorithm adding the input variable values together, as in Figure 9.5.

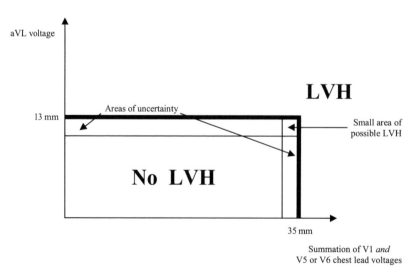

aVL voltage

13 mm

Areas of uncertainty

LVH

Small area of
possible LVH

No LVH

35 mm

Summation of V1 *and*
V5 or V6 chest lead voltages

Figure 9.9 Two lines are required to define the boundary between cases and non-cases according to these criteria. The small area where both criteria are almost met could be included in the LVH region by incorporating the algorithm in Figure 9.6.

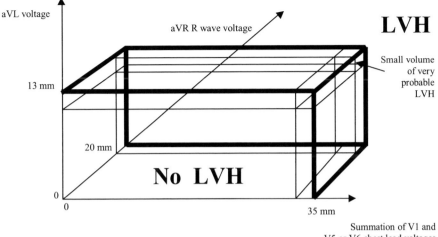

Figure 9.10   There are now three variable dimensions and the boundary between cases and non-cases is defined by three planes. A small volume is identified which includes cases that very nearly satisfy all three criteria (see text).

non-cases. The areas of uncertainty could be investigated by gathering more data in order to clarify the most appropriate position of the boundary, using the same model. The difficulty arises because there are potentially several combinations of values that could define useful decision boundaries. For instance, we could incorporate the small volume indicated in Figure 9.10 as a possible region of LVH cases by adding in three planes orthogonal to the existing decision planes.

Identifying patients at risk of coronary heart disease (CHD)

Suppose we wish to identify patients at highest risk of developing CHD in the next 10 years. Each risk variable could be searched separately (e.g. those patients with systolic blood pressure greater than 160 mmHg, OR those with diabetes, OR those greater than 70 years old), in combination (e.g. those with cholesterol over 5.0 mmol/l AND who smoke tobacco), or as a combined set of numerous such classes. Alternatively, we could define our target as the output of the Framingham algorithm[4] applied across the entire population. By doing this, we are using the Framingham equation not as a risk calculation tool for an individual patient (its traditional use), but as a *pattern recognition device for a population*. We have gone beyond the use of simple combinations of AND and OR to a search on the output of an algorithm that could in principle include non-linear terms through which a more complex decision boundary might be defined.

Box 9.1 describes a project undertaken in 1997 in a North Yorkshire general practice, in which a series of searches were carried out to identify patients requiring cholesterol measurement according to the Sheffield table criteria.[5] A final target group of 189 patients was identified by combining the results of 13 separate

Box 9.1   The Sheffield table survey 1997

The Sheffield tables were published in 1996, and consist of rows and columns of cells, each cell representing a combination of risk factor values (age, smoking status, diabetes status, hypertension status and LVH status). Separate tables are given for men and women. Each cell contains a cholesterol value at which that combination of risk factors would produce a risk of developing coronary heart disease (CHD) of $\geq 30\%$ in the next 10 years. The cholesterol values were obtained using the Framingham equation, an algorithm for calculating CHD risk. Many of the cells in the tables are empty – the cholesterol level would need to be so high to produce such a risk that no patient is likely to be so affected e.g. women less than 40 years with no risk factors.

These tables provide a framework for searching a practice population to identify candidates for cholesterol measurement. In 1997, a series of searches was carried out for this purpose on a North Yorkshire population. Because LVH status was frequently unknown or unrecorded, this was not included. The separate search protocols and results were:

Search	Sex	Hypertension	Smoking	Diabetes	Age range (years)	Result (number identified)
Sheffield 1	Male	Y	Y	Y	30–70	0
Sheffield 2	Male	Y	Y	N	34–70	12
Sheffield 3	Male	Y	N	Y	36–70	3
Sheffield 4	Male	Y	N	N	40–70	42
Sheffield 5	Male	N	Y	Y	48–70	1
Sheffield 6	Male	N	Y	N	54–70	29
Sheffield 7	Male	N	N	Y	58–70	3
Sheffield 8	Male	N	N	N	64–70	47
Sheffield 9	Female	Y	Y	Y	36–70	1
Sheffield 10	Female	Y	N	Y	40–70	3
Sheffield 11	Female	Y	Y	N	42–70	6
Sheffield 12	Female	Y	N	N	50–70	41
Sheffield 13	Female	N	Y	Y	52–70	1

As a result, a total of 189 patients were identified out of a population of 2137 patients. Their notes were then tagged electronically and each patient subsequently invited in for cholesterol measurement and, where it would then make a difference to treatment decisions, an ECG to determine LVH status.

searches. This involved a combination of AND and OR search operations on the database. However, the risk factors are all related through the Framingham algorithm, and so the algorithm itself could in principle have been used to identify the same subgroup of patients at potentially high risk of CHD. Such a search mechanism defines a pattern in a population by computing a function of multiple inputs extracted from the data. This technique is still not generally available in primary care in the UK.

More complex models

While most classification problems can be solved with linear models, some may require that more complex models be constructed. The higher 'complexity' of a model in this context is not necessarily just associated with the number of variables, but rather the characteristics of the functions that can be modelled. Consider as a very simple example the decision to recommend flu vaccines for those who are either very young (5 years or less) or elderly (65 years or more), provided there is no contraindication. Imagine we wish to develop a simple technique to produce recommendations by identifying suitable candidates using an algorithm similar to those in the figures above. Linear models cannot be used in this problem directly. Either a transformation has to be applied to the age variable (e.g. a quadratic transformation) or a non-linear classification model would have to be used. The problem is illustrated in Figure 9.11, which shows a network with one input (age) and a single output ('recommend vaccine'). Note that there is no way to adjust the weights and thresholds to obtain a correct recommendation for all ages (either the very young or the elderly will receive no recommendation).

If, however, two hidden nodes are added to this network, one firing for 'young' and another firing for 'old', then the correct recommendation can be given for these two age groups (Figure 9.12).

Neural networks with hidden nodes can therefore overcome the problem of linear inseparability, and may involve multiple input variables and more than one hidden layer. 'Training' of the network typically involves a process termed 'back propagation', in which the weights are initially given random values, but are then adjusted according to the differences between actual and target outputs (the *error*) as input patterns from a training set of cases/non-cases are presented to the network.[6]

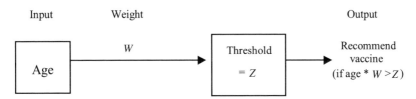

Figure 9.11   There is no linear range of weight values for W which will be positive for both low and high age values but not for intermediate ages, so this model cannot produce satisfactory recommendations for both the young and old without some sort of non-linear transformation. The problem is linearly inseparable.

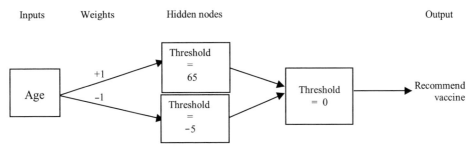

Figure 9.12   A layer of hidden nodes overcomes the problem by including separate nodes, one of which fires at high age values and the other at low age values.

In determining the structure of a classification boundary, a neural network with sufficient hidden nodes can define an unlimited number of linear or non-linear boundary features[2] in order to improve the specificity and sensitivity in the regions of uncertainty, and can also identify isolated regions of the space that are disconnected from the main region where most cases exist.[7] Such isolated regions might exist in classification problems where interactions between multiple variables are important. Neural networks are particularly useful (and superior to alternative techniques) in the case of 'Exclusive/Or' problems, where a class is defined by membership of one category or another, but *not* both. 'Exclusive/Or' presented an obstacle to neural network research in the 1960s,[8] an obstacle now known to be solved with hidden nodes. A great advance to the field in the 1980s was the publication of the backpropagation algorithm to determine weights connecting to and from the hidden nodes.

Neural networks have now been used in numerous areas of healthcare,[9] including the clinical diagnosis of common medical conditions, radiological interpretation, outcome prediction following surgery and resuscitation, and in the interpretation of electroencephalograms. They provide a more flexible way of recognising interactions between input variables compared to logistic regression. Publishing bias may account to some extent for the apparent success of these techniques in the literature, but there are numerous examples of their use in difficult classification problems. Box 9.2 gives an example of the use of a neural network in the diagnosis of acute myocardial infarction (AMI) in patients presenting with chest pain to an emergency department in Sweden.

Box 9.2   Neural network diagnosis of acute myocardial infarction

The potential benefits of neural networks over simpler interpretation techniques was demonstrated by Heden *et al.* in the journal *Circulation* in 1997.[10] This group compared the ability of a neural network to diagnose AMI from ECGs with that of simpler 'rule-based' approaches (similar to that described above for diagnosing LVH), and also with assessments made by an experienced cardiologist.

The study population involved ECGs taken on patients presenting with chest pain to an emergency department in Lund, Sweden, between 1990 and 1995. A total of 1120 ECGs from patients with AMI were studied, as well as 10 452 control ECGs from patients in whom AMI was excluded or who were not then admitted to hospital. The neural network used 72 input variable measurements from each ECG. The network contained 11 nodes in the hidden layer. The synapse weights were initially set at random values, and then adjusted during training by back propagation using outcome data. Cross-validation was obtained by dividing the dataset into subgroups, which took turns in training and testing. This was necessary to avoid 'over-training', in which network error increases after reaching a minimum value.

The specificity and sensitivity of the neural network for diagnosing AMI significantly exceeded that of both the rule-based computer interpretations and the cardiologist.

Other solutions to the problem of linear inseparability

In the above example of vaccination, the researcher knows the influence of age in the final recommendation. We specify our own definition of the patient groups we wish to include in the recommendation. In other problems, however, these relationships may not be known, but we may still be able to construct models that are able to classify cases into known categories (even though the precise definition of the determining profiles may not be as easily interpretable). In real-world pattern recognition classification problems such as the identification of patients who are at risk for coronary disease, not only is there a large number of variables to consider, but again the possibility of linear inseparability of the data (as in the example above). As explained before, linear inseparability in a multivariate space means that there is no simple point that can separate cases using a single variable, no single line that can separate cases using two variables, no single plane that can separate cases using three variables, and so on. Figure 9.13 illustrates this concept for two variables. On the x axis, we depict the variable 'age', and on the y axis, we depict 'contraindication'. The point (0,0) means (young, no contraindication), the point (1,1) corresponds to a patient who is (middle-aged, contraindication), while the point (2,1) corresponds to (elderly, contraindication). By using these two variables, we can define six categories of patients, two of which should be given the flu shot: the ones represented by (0,0) and (2,0). All others should not receive the shot. Note that these points cannot be separated from the others using a single line (two lines are required). This is a simplified example of a non-linearly separable problem. This type of problem cannot be modelled using linear models such as logistic regression (unless variable transformations or variable interactions are added, which requires domain knowledge, since an exhaustive search for all possible variable combinations is usually prohibitive in real-world problems).

There are several types of models that can deal with non-linearly separable data. Neural networks with hidden nodes, discussed above, are one example. Others

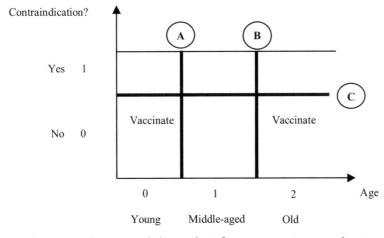

Figure 9.13 Separation of recommended cases for influenza vaccination according to age and presence or absence of a contraindication. The solid lines A, B and C correspond to the decision boundaries.

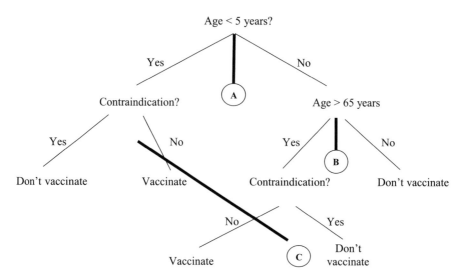

Figure 9.14   A regression tree defining the boundaries for influenza immunisation based on age and presence or absence of a contraindication.

include classification and regression trees,[11] and support vector machines with non-linear kernels.[12]

Classification and regression trees

Classification and regression trees, also known as decision trees, or recursive partitioning models, allow for non-linear separation of cases. Figure 9.13 shows how the lines marked A, B and C would separate the cases recommended for flu shots from the others. Figure 9.14 shows a regression tree corresponding to this model. Each branch of the tree corresponds to the separation of the cases according to a single variable. The leaves of the tree correspond to areas in Figure 9.13. The rules determining the decision can be 'read' from the tree, by following a case from the root to the corresponding leaf.

Support vector machines

Support vector machines are another alternative for classification of linearly inseparable cases. In this model, there is a kernel function whose objective is to 'fold' the space such that the problem becomes linearly separable and can be solved by a linear classifier that is determined according to the 'support vectors', or characteristics of the cases and non-cases that lie at the decision boundary. (See Figures 9.15 and 9.16.)

   Returning to the issue of coronary heart disease risk, Figure 9.17 uses a similar system of weights and thresholds to the ECG interpretation device described above, modelling the Framingham algorithm as a synapse, based on an example of weight values in a 55-year-old male individual taken from a published source.[13] Note that the summation of the weight values (21) falls short of the threshold of 30 traditionally recognised as 'high risk' (i.e. 30% risk of developing coronary heart disease in the next 10 years), a threshold currently used in the UK for rationing lipid-lowering drug therapy in primary prevention.[14] This does not mean that the patient requires no advice or follow up for his risk factors. The Framingham Heart

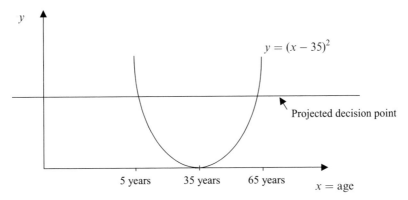

Figure 9.15   The quadratic function $y = (x - 35)^2$ effectively folds the age axis at the midway point between the recommended age boundaries to allow a single linear classifier. In the transformed space, still represented in one dimension (the y axis), it is possible to construct a linear classifier of $n - 1$ dimensions (a point) to separate cases from non-cases. The support vectors are the case and non-case that are closest and equidistant to the point. They define the decision boundary.

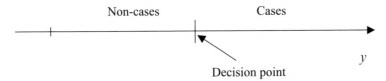

Figure 9.16   Represented as a single axis, the quadratic kernel function allows a single point to distinguish cases from non-cases. More complex functions could perform similar transformations in higher-dimensional spaces.

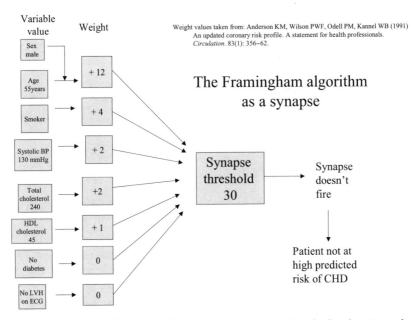

Figure 9.17   The Framingham algorithm as a synapse, recognising high-risk patterns for CHD (cholesterol values are given in mg/dl in the published source).

Study[4] was undertaken in the 1940s–1970s, and since then a number of interventions relevant to cardiovascular outcomes have become part of routine care. It is therefore likely that the study's predictions may become outdated over time. A different algorithm is now used for patients with diabetes based on UKPDS (United Kingdom Prospective Diabetes Study) data, which takes account of other factors relevant to CHD risk, including duration of diabetes and degree of glycaemia.[15] These factors were not included in the Framingham model, whose cohort included only 337 patients with diabetes.

When viewed as a synapse, it becomes possible to appreciate how such an algorithm might be adapted through the emergence of new research evidence, by the inclusion of more input variables, the establishment of more interactions between the risk factors, and the adjustment of weight and threshold values. This creates the opportunity for applying more complex models to the problem, capable of recognising more adequately the interactive nature of its components. A hidden layer applied to Figure 9.17, for instance, might enable clusters or subclasses of input variables within the profile to influence predictions if appropriate, and so potentially improve predictive performance.

Summary

This chapter has explored some of the techniques through which patterns in healthcare datasets may be recognised and interpreted. While most classification problems lend themselves well to linear modelling, the increasing availability of clinical and genetic data and the recognition of interactions between multiple input variables may enable more complex strategies to assist clinicians in tailoring care appropriately to the needs of individual patients. This may then lead to more efficient case detection in the population, improved prediction of outcomes in situations of high uncertainty and a more satisfactory picture of disease risk factor profiles.

Acknowledgement

The authors thank Staal Vinterbo for his helpful suggestions.

References

1 Gray DP, Steele R, Sweeney K *et al.* (1994) Generalists in medicine. *BMJ.* **308**: 486–7.
2 Kattan M (2002) Statistical prediction models, artificial neural networks, and the sophism 'I am a patient, not a statistic'. *J Clin Oncol.* **20**: 885–7.
3 Julian DG (1988) *Cardiology* (5e). Baillière Tindall, London.
4 Kannel WB, McGee D, Gordon T (1976) A general cardiovascular risk profile: the Framingham Study. *Am J Cardiol.* **38**: 46–51.
5 Ramsey LE, Haq IU, Jackson PR *et al.* (1996) The Sheffield table for primary prevention of coronary heart disease: corrected. *Lancet.* **348**: 1251–2.
6 Bishop CM (1995) *Neural Networks for Pattern Recognition.* Oxford University Press, Oxford.

7   Cross SS, Harrison RF, Lee Kennedy R (1995) Introduction to neural networks. *Lancet*. **346**: 1075–79.

8   Flake GW (1998) *The Computational Beauty of Nature*. MIT Press, Cambridge, MA.

9   Baxt WG (1995) Application of neural networks to clinical medicine. *Lancet*. **346**: 1135–8.

10 Heden B, Ohlin H, Rittner R *et al.* (1997) Acute myocardial infarction detected in the 12-lead ECG by artificial neural networks. *Circulation*. **96**(6): 1798–1802.

11 Breiman L, Friedman J, Olshen RA *et al.* (1984) *Classification and Regression Trees*. Chapman and Hall, Boca Raton, FL.

12 Boser BE, Guyon IM, Vapnik VN (1992) *A training algorithm for optimal margin classifiers*. In: D Haussler (ed.) *Proceedings of the 5th Annual ACM Workshop on Computational Learning Theory*, pp. 144–152. ACM Press, New York.

13 Anderson KM, Wilson PWF, Odell PM *et al.* (1991) An updated coronary risk profile. A statement for health professionals. *Circulation*. **83**(1): 356–62.

14 Department of Health (2000) *National Service Framework: coronary heart disease*. Chapter Two: Preventing coronary heart disease in high-risk patients. DoH, London.

15 Stevens RJ, Kothari V, Adler AI *et al.* (2001) The UKPDS risk engine: a model for the risk of coronary heart disease in Type II diabetes (UKPDS 56). *Clinical Science*. **101**(6): 671–9.

CHAPTER 10

Adaptation to changing landscapes in clinical care

Tim Holt

As we have outlined earlier in this book, complex adaptive systems are able to make internal adjustments in response to changing patterns in the environment and so learn adaptively. As time goes by, current behaviour is then determined not only by what is happening in the immediate environment, but also by historical patterns established over a longer timescale.

Collective human behaviour is the result of a complex process of adaptation that involves three basic phases of learning:

1   Learning through the unique experiences of individuals gained within the time-scale of a lifetime.
2   Social conditioning resulting from the cultural norms and beliefs of the wider community developed over many generations and perpetuated through teaching, cultural practices, and sharing of information through books, journals and (in more recent times) electronic sources.
3   Genetically determined behaviour, resulting from a long period of evolutionary history through which our genes have become adapted to a changing environment.

Organisational learning

If we regard the health service as a complex adaptive system, then we might recognise these phases in our everyday practice. How does the system as a whole 'learn'? How can we enable the past experiences of the system (which may be above the level of any individual 'agent') to influence current behaviour in a productive way?

The first phase is exemplified in clinical care through the relationship that develops over time between a practitioner and a patient or client, and is discussed by Andrew Innes in Chapter 3. This is a powerful determinant that is often undervalued in the effort to streamline clinical behaviour. It is a source of flexibility at the clinical interface, which allows the patient's narrative to be set in the context of the clinician–patient relationship. In a sense, this relationship moves continuously as a unique trajectory through time, but in another sense the system as a whole has thousands of such trajectories running in parallel as relationships between practitioners and patients develop.

The second phase of learning has been explored by Paul Robinson in Chapter 7. This involves the influence of research evidence and consensus opinion over clinical behaviour and patient choices. As we have seen, this process is a complex one given the multidimensional and interconnected nature of patients' and clinicians' knowledge, beliefs, expectations and receptiveness. It is not surprising that in clinical contexts phase two is highly dependent on phase one.

The third phase of system learning involves aspects of clinical behaviour that change over longer time periods, due not to our changing knowledge of individual patients, nor because the nature of a disease process has become more adequately researched, but because of actual changes in the disease process or pattern itself. Examples might be the changes in patterns of immunological disorders, malignancy or cardiovascular risk during the twentieth century. Such effects may result from changes in nutritional status, social variables such as housing and sanitation, gene flow between patient populations, medical interventions and countless other factors. Past research may then no longer be applicable to our current patients, not because the conclusions were incorrect at the time, but because the patients or the diseases themselves have changed. To pick a topical example, consider the association between hormone replacement therapy (HRT) use and risk of breast cancer.[1] The initiation of HRT in a patient might be determined by the information provided by her clinician and set in the context of their relationship, her own beliefs and her other sources of advice (phase 1), current research- and opinion-based knowledge reflecting up-to-date thinking on the risk of breast cancer with HRT use (phase 2), and finally, the actual association between breast cancer and HRT use, which may itself vary over time (phase 3).

How can such longer-term changes be detected, monitored and allowed to influence clinical behaviour appropriately into the indefinite future? A novel approach that is now becoming possible and which very much resonates with the theme of adaptive learning in CAS, would be to allow the outcomes of past clinical behaviour to feed back on current behaviour via electronic record keeping. This is the theme of this final chapter.

Adapting our clinical behaviour in response to recorded data

The development of large integrated clinical databases is changing the way that we approach data collection, and creates opportunities for allowing the results of what we do to influence and inform future clinical behaviour. This represents a novel mechanism through which research data might be gathered and 'best practice' determined. For example, 2003 saw the start of the QRESEACH programme, based at the University of Nottingham, which pools anonymised information from general practices throughout the UK and makes it available for medical research.[2] How might such combined databases be explored using some of the principles outlined in this book, to ensure that care is more, and not less, sensitively tailored to the needs of individuals?

The first step will not only be to recognise the database's *structure*, but also its *dynamics*. Large databases derived from cohort studies such as the Framingham Heart Study,[3] represent a fixed volume of information that is there for anyone to examine at any future date, but will not necessarily remain valid indefinitely, particularly as new developments such as novel drug therapies are developed, and new risk factors (including genetic markers) are discovered. One of the advantages of integrated database research (apart from the sheer volume of data available) is that the system is an ongoing, 'living' representation of how we work, what we find and what we do.

Landscapes in multidimensional space

To recap on an important theme of the last chapter: complex pattern recognition involves not only the retrieval of data on multiple variables, but also the construction of *algorithms* that use the variables as inputs and produce outputs that define patterns, classify cases or make predictions.

The concept of a *space of possible values* of the numerous variables in a system, discussed in Part One, has been a recurrent theme in this book, providing a general framework for modelling the structure and dynamics of complex systems. I would like now to expand on this idea and discuss the related concept of a *landscape*, a model familiar to population biologists and now an important tool in complexity theory.

Imagine a protein made up of a sequence of amino acids, responsible for catalysing a biochemical reaction. The protein exists in a 'space' of possible sequences, a space with multiple dimensions, because at each position in the molecule there is a range of around 20 or so possible amino acids. An individual protein (such as trypsin or bradykinin) exists at a *single position* in this space, and a change or mutation affecting one or more amino acids will alter the protein's position in 'sequence space'.

If we define 'fitness' as the protein's efficiency as a catalyst (and this is of course only a small factor in the wider sense of *fitness* of the entire organism[4]), then each amino acid makes a contribution to the protein's 'fitness'. However, this contribution is utterly dependent on the other amino acids present, because a lone amino acid has no catalytic properties itself. Some functions of proteins may be highly dependent on the particular amino acid occupying a specific location in the peptide chain. Mutation affecting this amino acid may be seriously detrimental, while other mutations may not affect the protein's function at all. When we think of the 'sequence space' of possible proteins, certain positions have high fitness, while others (often close by, sometimes literally 'next door') have zero fitness – the protein at this position has no functional activity. Inborn errors of metabolism involving single amino acid mutations may have disastrous effects, threatening the viability of the whole organism.

So the 'fitness' of an individual amino acid has little or no meaning, but each position in protein sequence space can be assigned a fitness value for catalysing this particular reaction in this particular context. Fitness can then be plotted as an additional axis in the space, to produce a *fitness landscape*.

Fitness landscapes were first described by the population biologist Sewall Wright in the 1930s, but have since then been studied extensively by theorists such as Stuart Kauffman.[4] Biological evolution involves an exploration of fitness landscapes, in which differential survival of variant individuals leads to the population moving over time up fitness gradients towards local or global optima (Figure 10.1).

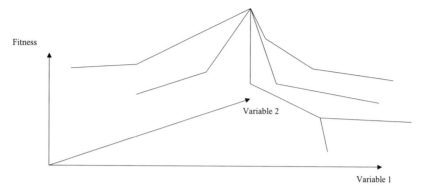

Figure 10.1 A fitness landscape involving two variables. In principle, any number of variables could be included. In this case there is a single global maximum fitness value, roughly corresponding to mid-range values of the two variables. More 'rugged' landscapes may exist where there are local maxima with lower fitness than the global maximum.

Risk landscapes

By analogy to fitness, the *risk of a particular disease* is in a sense a function of an individual's risk factors, in which the significance of a single factor is determined partly by the context defined by the others, so it might be useful to plot overall risk as an axis in risk factor space (Figures 10.2 and 10.3). The resulting *risk landscapes* could then be studied in a similar way to the fitness landscapes of population biology.

Risk landscapes are now an established tool in risk modification programmes (even though they are not usually labelled as such). The charts published by the Joint British Societies are risk landscapes, where two risk factors at a time are plotted, and risk itself given as a colour with gradients of increasing risk across the chart.[5]

Figure 10.3 illustrates a condition in which there is an 'island' of increased risk surrounded by lower risk areas. Remember that these diagrams can only portray two risk factors at a time. The risk landscape may in principle be constructed using

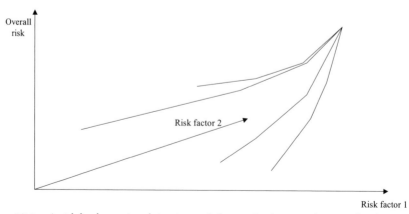

Figure 10.2 A risk landscape involving two risk factors. In this case the overall risk continues to rise with increasing values for each of the two risk factor variables. The peak value for overall risk is the position where both the variables are at a maximum.

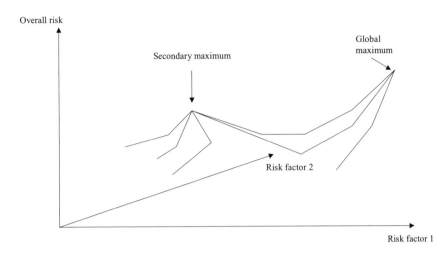

Figure 10.3   A risk landscape for a condition in which there is a secondary local maximum value for overall risk, surrounded by lower risk areas, in the 'foothills' of the landscape's global maximum.

as many risk factors as are relevant, with each position (combination of risk variable values) associated with its own level of overall risk.

What determines the structure of landscapes?

Some landscapes appear to be 'rugged,' with multiple secondary maxima, while others are relatively smooth. Stuart Kauffman has studied this property extensively, and describes a spectrum of patterns, starting with the smooth single peaked 'Mount Fujiama' (similar to that represented in Figure 10.1), through more gentler rolling landscapes, to the rugged 'Alps' environment in which the 'surface' may be so rugged as to be *uncorrelated* – two nearby points on the landscape are no more likely to be similar in fitness than more distantly separated points. Kauffman has developed a simplified model of interaction between the components, which he calls *NK landscapes*, [3] mentioned in Chapter 1. In this model, N is the number of components (amino acids in a protein, genes in a genotype, etc.), and K is the number of other components that influence the fitness contribution of each component. The degree of interaction between components can therefore be tuned by varying the K parameter.

Kauffman's studies show that the structure of NK landscapes is highly dependent on the degree of interaction, K. Even systems with large numbers of components (high values of N) will be smooth if K is zero. The next question becomes: how interconnected are real-life systems, and can this insight be applied to disease risk profiles?

It may at first seem unlikely that a multipeaked risk landscape could represent a human disease. It might be assumed that risk factors (particularly continuous risk variables such as cholesterol or systolic blood pressure) follow a spectrum from low, through medium to high risk. Even if the relationship between the value of the risk factor and the risk it confers is non-linear, how can it produce a secondary maximum like the one in Figure 10.3? But the risk gradient of many diseases reverses as age increases, such as testicular cancer, which is commoner in the third and fourth decades than in children or the elderly, and asthma, which is commoner in children and the elderly than in young adults. Markers such as haemoglobin or potassium levels, as well as dietary factors such as sodium intake, produce the same effect of risk gradient reversal so that, as discussed in Chapter 9, the highest risk groups are *not linearly separable*. The 'J-shaped curve' relating alcohol consumption to CHD risk is another well-known example. Such relationships would produce a 'ripple' in the risk landscape, and if more than one such risk factor were involved, a hillock or depression might appear. As we recognise increasing numbers of risk factors, including genetic markers, it becomes more likely that, particularly where the interactions between them are important, the smoothness of the landscape would be disrupted by secondary maxima or minima.

So how and why is this model useful? The first answer would be that the identification of 'islands' of increased risk challenges our intuitive impression of disease predisposition as a simple summation of risk factors. Just as we may identify local risk peaks, we might also be able to recognise local *minima*, in which a certain combination of risk factors has a lower risk than surrounding regions. Risk modification (which, when successful involves movement down risk gradients) might then be achieved most effectively by identifying a realistically achievable nearby local minimum for the patient, which might be much 'closer' in the landscape than the global minimum risk position.

Even where there are no secondary maxima and the risk landscape is smooth (as in Figure 10.2), a knowledge of its structure may still be useful in determining the easiest way 'downwards', and also the most cost-effective way downwards. An example of this would be the finding that the majority of patients at high risk of coronary heart disease could have their overall risk reduced as much by stopping smoking as by taking lipid-lowering medication.[6] This was a factor in fuelling the move to make nicotine replacement therapy available on prescription in the UK. It was a funding decision based partly on the topography of the CHD risk landscape.

The space of possible weight values

Now imagine that instead of plotting a risk landscape using risk factor variable values on each axis, we construct a *space of possible weight values* for a pattern recognition or prediction algorithm. Each axis in the space represents a range of weights for each input variable value, and the algorithm itself occupies a single point in this space.

Just as patients move, during their lives, through a space of possible risk factor values, each position carrying its own overall risk level, so a prediction algorithm can be allowed to move through a space of possible weight values, each position associated with a level of performance for the algorithm in terms of its ability to recognise patterns or predict outcomes.

A prediction algorithm might be 'trained' by exposure to a database containing information on risk factors and later development of the disease, or symptom profiles and diagnostic outcomes, and from this data the most appropriate initial weights could be determined (defining its position in the space of possible weight combinations.) This position in a sense determines the *'fitness'* of the algorithm − its

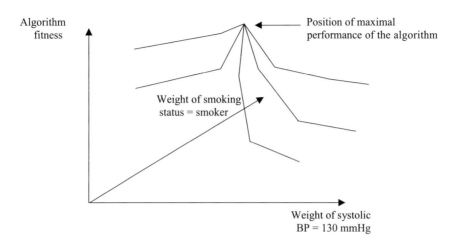

Algorithm
fitness

Position of maximal
performance of the algorithm

Weight of smoking
status = smoker

Weight of systolic
BP = 130 mmHg

Figure 10.4   Possible fitness landscape of a prediction algorithm for coronary heart disease risk, indicating the global optimum position. Only two of the many risk factor values can be included in this three-dimensional reconstruction.

predictive performance, its ability (forgive the pun) to provide the best statistical *fit* between predicted and actual outcomes. In seeking the best sequence of weight values, we are looking for the maximum value for the algorithm's fitness, the global optimum position, the peak in the landscape (Figure 10.4).

This process of exploration, through which peaks of predictive accuracy are sought, is very reminiscent of the process described above, through which biological populations move 'uphill' through fitness landscapes towards maxima. However, evolving organisms are restricted, for at least two reasons, in the way they can move through a fitness landscape. First of all, they can only move, in genetic terms, in fairly small steps. Large, 'hopeful' jumps through the landscape are unlikely to be successful, as intermediate stages in evolution must all be viable (and fertile). While the mutation of a number of genes may improve fitness more than a single gene mutation, locating viable, fitter variants through 'macromutation' involving many gene loci at once (representing large jumps in sequence space) gets increasingly unlikely the further from the starting position we go.[7] Second, they tend to move *upwards* along fitness gradients, and may get stuck on small local peaks surrounded by regions of lower fitness. This phenomenon explains some of the less than ideal design features in nature, where a structure or functional process has evolved that is too far away from fitter alternatives in the landscape for evolution to reach them without intermediate steps that are less fit. The more variables involved, the more likely it is that there will be an uphill 'escape route' from any position,[8] but the risk of getting stuck at a local maximum still remains. (Mark Ridley's standard text *Evolution*[9] gives a fascinating discussion on this, but the details are beyond our current requirements in this book.)

Computer software might be similarly constrained, and a number of possible ways of exploring the weight space of a prediction algorithm are possible. Clearly such a space, when it involves multiple axes, is vast. How might we explore this space in as efficient a manner as possible to arrive at positions of high performance for the algorithm? There are a number of options:

1   Using our data and an algorithm involving weighted inputs, we could calcu-
    late the predictive accuracy of every position in the algorithm's weight space.
    However, for multiple input variables this would be very time-consuming and
    inefficient even for a powerful computer, and most positions produce very
    poor predictions (just as the majority of amino acid combinations have no
    catalytic activity).
2   We could conduct a 'walk' through the space by randomly mutating the algo-
    rithm, starting at a likely looking position we might select using a previous
    dataset. Each new position might then be assessed to determine how closely it
    fits the data (and therefore how predictively powerful the algorithm at this
    position was). However, unless the walk was designed to proceed upwards
    along fitness gradients, the accuracy would almost certainly fall off rapidly with
    each mutated step. A walk up local fitness gradients might improve accuracy in
    the short term but would risk getting 'stuck' on a local maximum that might be
    considerably inferior to the global maximum. This risk would relate to the
    'ruggedness' and degree of correlation of the landscape.
3   We could arrange for individual algorithms to 'breed' with each other. Variants
    of the initial algorithm would be produced, as in biological species, either by
    'cross-over' of two 'parent' algorithms or by mutation, and then be selected
    according to their performance in a way reminiscent of natural selection –
    a process in which the better performing algorithms 'survive' and breed at a
    higher rate at the expense of less 'fit' variants. In this way, the landscape is
    explored through the differential survival of variants of the initial positions.
    This is the mechanism on which *genetic algorithms* are based.[10]

Genetic algorithms

How in practice would such 'breeding' occur? Let's first of all recap on what
happens when a real biological gene is replicated. A string of purine and pyridine
bases (A, G, T and C) makes up a DNA sequence. Each base is linked to its fellow
base in an adjacent string, forming a string of pairs:

AACGTACGTCAGTCAGCT
TTGCATGCAGTCAGTCGA

Because A always pairs with T, and G with C, the adjacent string is specified by
the first string, so that we can consider just one base sequence on its own:

AACGTACGTCAGTCAGCT

Imagine now that the organism is to reproduce sexually. Each gene sequence in
the organism's chromosomes has two slightly different copies, one from each of its
parents. During meiosis (the process through which the gametes are produced)
segments in these adjacent strings may *cross over*, in this example at a point five
bases in from the left, indicated by the underline:

<u>AACGT</u>ACGTCAGTCAGCT   Parent sequence 1
<u>AATGG</u>ACGTCAGACAGCT   Parent sequence 2

producing two daughter strings:

AATGGACGTCAGTCAGCT

and

AACGTACGTCAGACAGCT

Neither of these daughter strings is the same as either of the 'parents', but the jump has involved not a *random* mutation of five bases, but the cutting and pasting (literally, as I prepare this manuscript) of an intact sequence of bases which were *functionally coherent* in the parent string. This allows bold, but not hopeless, jumps to occur in sequence space during the process of replication and provides the most important source of variation in sexually reproducing species. It allows the fitness landscape to be explored in a much more productive way than random mutation would alone, making it less likely that the population will get trapped on a local fitness maximum or that the daughter sequences are so different as to be unviable. Computer algorithms can of course 'breed' at extremely fast rates and can if necessary 'cross' individual parent algorithms separated distantly in the landscape.

Breeding the Framingham algorithm

How could this process be applied to a prediction algorithm? Genetic algorithms are only one of many possible ways to train or retrain such an algorithm, but are worth discussing here as an example of software adaptation. All algorithms, like software programs in general, can be described by a sequence of binary digital bits (0 or 1). So the Framingham algorithm, including the equation's coefficients, could be similarly described. But in order to make it easier to visualise, let's imagine the algorithm as a string of values for the weights associated with each of the input variables, using the values given in Figure 9.17 in Chapter 9 (p. 145):

Table 10.1   The Framingham algorithm as a string of weight values

	Sex	Age (years)	Smoking status	Systolic BP	Total cholesterol	HDL cholesterol	Diabetes status	LVH status
Values	Male	55	Smoker	130	240	45	No	No
Weights in the example cited[II]		+12	+4	+2	+2	+1	0	0
Possible variant algorithms								
Alternative weights		+10	+5	+2	+3	+1	0	−1
Another alternative		+11	+6	+1	+4	+2	−1	−1

While the string would need to include weight values for all possible input variable values (and most of these would be non-applicable to any one individual patient), it becomes possible to see the algorithm as a long string of values which could be varied not simply by adjusting one or two of the weights randomly (as in the variants above), but by crossing over an entire segment of the sequence in the same way as in the gene sequence example described earlier. The algorithms could then produce a number of 'daughters', any of which might be superior to its parents in terms of predictive performance.

Combining examples 1 and 2 above through cross-over at position 3:

$$+10 \quad +5 \quad +2 \quad +2 \quad +1 \quad 0 \quad 0$$

Combining examples 2 and 3 above through cross-over at position 4:

$$+11 \quad +6 \quad +1 \quad +4 \quad +1 \quad 0 \quad -1$$

New sequences could then be assessed by measuring the predictive performance of the variant algorithms using a large database containing input variables and outcomes, and the more successful algorithms could then be allowed to breed faster than their inferior competitors. As a result, a process of Darwinian selection would allow the algorithms to search the landscape and ultimately find the optimal fitness position. An advantage of this approach is that any changes in the landscape itself over time (due to changes in the relationship between risk factor patterns and CHD development) could be tracked. The genetic algorithm would continuously evolve inside its own software environment by adapting to a moving landscape.

Remember Pikaia, our little Burgess shale ancestor mentioned in Chapter 1? For a visual demonstration of a genetic algorithm exploring a complex landscape, visit the PIKAIA program at www.hao.ucar.edu/public/research/si/pikaia/pikaia.html

The space of possible interactions between the weights

So far, this discussion has described the way a genetic algorithm might evolve through a space of possible weight values. But depending on the model used, there is more to such an algorithm than simply its weight values. Just as the *amino acid sequence* of a protein does not necessarily specify the protein's secondary and tertiary structure (structure that results from *interactions* between the amino acids and is essential to its catalytic properties), this framework has not so far allowed the *interactions* between the variables to be adequately represented. How might these interactions be modelled, in such a way that the various possible patterns of interaction could be similarly explored in a search for optimal performance?

One solution would be to model the interactions using the neural network design discussed in Chapter 9, using not only inputs and outputs but also one or more *hidden layers*. The structure of the network might then be defined using parameters such as the number of elements in each hidden layer, or the number of connections between one layer and the next. Alternatives (laid out again using binary digits) could 'breed' with each other to evolve the best network structure in terms of predictive performance. This approach combines some of the benefits of neural networks and genetic algorithms, and has been elegantly demonstrated in a paper by Dybowski *et al.* in the *Lancet* in 1996.[12] This group used the principle described above to allow variant neural network algorithms to evolve towards an optimum structure through random cross-over and mutation followed by differential survival favouring the 'fittest' variants. In this case, the neural network had been designed to predict outcomes in an intensive care unit using 18 inputs that defined the patient's condition, medical history and demographic profile. The variants differed in the structure of the hidden layers (see Chapter 9), and after seven 'generations' the fittest variants converged towards an optimal structure that failed to improve in subsequent generations. A peak in the neural network's fitness landscape had been reached.

Adapting to a changing landscape

How might the continual tracking of database landscapes help us in the delivery of clinical care? The algorithms that determine the structure of the landscapes (such as the Framingham algorithm, at present our best model for the CHD risk landscape) represent a form of *memory*, a highly compressed representation of the information in the data. Even if the data from which the algorithm is initially trained are not kept on record forever, the algorithms themselves, rather like the DNA in our genes, have the potential to survive indefinitely over successive generations of patient and clinician. But changes in the structure of the landscape are likely to occur as discussed above, through both genetic and environmental influences. In the case of CHD risk, we are not so much dealing with a fixed landscape but a dynamic surface like that of the sea, which changes over time, albeit gradually. If we are to expect our prediction algorithms to still be useful in coming decades, then the evolution of the landscapes needs to result in adjustment to the internal parameters of the algorithms that represent them.

The possibility of tracking such changes in the combined national database of UK primary care has been discussed by myself and Lucila Ohno-Machado.[13] This would involve the linkage of databases from many participating practices committed to high-quality data collection and the use of a prediction algorithm able both to target patients requiring treatment and to identify areas of insufficient data in those at potentially high risk. In fact, in line with the recommendations of the UK's CHD National Service Framework,[14] this mechanism arises naturally through processes already in common practice through which patients who currently do not have CHD but who may be at high risk are identified and invited in to have their risk variables updated and their risk clarified. Figure 10.5 outlines the model as suggested in our paper, and could in principle be applied to other areas of care (including, as mentioned above, the identification of symptom complexes suggesting malignancy). But of all the pattern recognition problems we face in primary care, the identification of individuals at high risk of CHD is unique, because a prediction algorithm is programmed into the computer software used by clinicians all over the UK, and outcomes (dates of onset of subsequent CHD development) are recorded within the same system, as are the input data. This opens up the possibility for allowing other factors to become included in the risk calculation, and for the adoption of more complex pattern recognition techniques, including

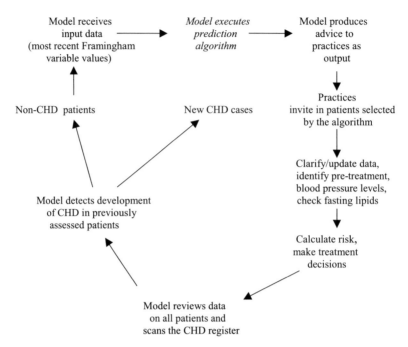

Figure 10.5 A nationwide adaptive prediction tool for coronary heart disease prevention.[13] The outcomes of the predictions are allowed to modify the algorithm, if necessary, by comparing input patterns with outcomes in both CHD and non-CHD cases.

neural networks. Such techniques have been applied to CHD risk assessment problems in the past,[15,16] but not using primary care databases. These techniques might allow a wider range of risk factors to be included, interactions between them to influence predictions, and, in the long run, the flexibility to adapt to changing risk patterns as they evolve over time. The use of alternative statistical models would enable the algorithm to be tailored to the available data, which in practice may often be incomplete for an individual patient.

Problems with this approach

Clearly such a system is highly dependent on the quality of the data available, and there have been concerns about this quality from the very beginning of electronic record keeping. However, there is evidence that data quality is improving, and this trend should hopefully continue as recording becomes increasingly standardised, particularly in areas such as chronic disease management.

Changes to the prediction algorithm will only be appropriate if the corresponding changes in the landscape are statistically significant rather than due to random fluctuation. The flexibility of the algorithm would need to be tuned to account for this and in practice this may create considerable difficulties. Cross *et al.* discuss this issue in the context of 'continuing education' following the initial training of neural networks.[17]

A further issue is that the Framingham algorithm is designed to make predictions on the basis of blood pressure and cholesterol levels taken *prior* to treatment.

We do not have a similar algorithm that uses treated levels as inputs, and yet many of the patients we assess in primary prevention contexts are already on treatment, at least for blood pressure. Clinicians tend to get round this problem either by identifying pre-treatment levels from the patient's record (measurements often taken many years beforehand and therefore unsatisfactory), or by using treated levels as inputs but then simply 'factoring in' an unspecified mark-up in the final estimate of risk in a treated patient. However, the ability of search techniques to distinguish patients who were, or were not on such medication when the measurement was taken means that, over time, a similar algorithm could in principle be developed that took account of this factor. Indeed, one of the attractions of this model is that it might enable such information to be recovered from modern populations, whose risk profiles, treatment histories and individual diversity are now extremely complex.

Testing the usefulness of the model

The model described above produces a number of research questions, which could readily be explored in primary care.

1   The patients identified by the model should have a higher average calculated risk of CHD than those identified using the strategy recommended in the NSF – namely, those with diagnosed hypertension and diabetes. The number needed to screen[18] (NNS) to find a case with greater than 30% 10-year risk should be consistently lower using the proposed model. If confirmed, this would demonstrate the model's greater efficiency at case recognition.
2   Over a period of years, the predictive performance of variant algorithms could be compared, based on recorded outcomes, with the Framingham algorithm to determine whether the adaptive modifications had improved the identification of those likely to develop CHD.
3   Advice to practices over which patients to invite in for screening would ultimately originate from the data of contemporary primary care, rather than from a past cohort study separated in time and place from the clinician and the patient. This might foster a feeling of *ownership* of the information, and greater confidence that it was genuinely applicable to the current practice population. This confidence should be demonstrable through surveys of clinicians' opinions over how welcome and useful this advice is in practice.

Summary

A hallmark feature of complex adaptive systems is their ability to *process information*, and learn from past experience. In clinical care, this happens through the unique relationships between clinicians and patients, through the process by which research evidence and consensus opinion influence clinical behaviour and patient choices, and through the detection of changes in the patterns of risk and disease at the population level. This chapter has explored the ways that complex modelling might improve the flexibility of clinical care delivery by recognising the interactive patterns of clinical variables and their dynamical evolution over time. Such models may allow us to more adequately assess not only the needs of individuals, but also the quality of care provision at the population level. The availability of information from large, integrated primary care databases may, if data quality becomes adequate, provide a new means through which difficult and complex research questions might be addressed.

References

1 Griffiths F (2003) Taking hormone replacement therapy. *BMJ*. **327**: 820–1.
2 www.nottingham.ac.uk/~mczqres/index.html
3 Kannel WB, McGee D, Gordon T (1976) A general cardiovascular risk profile: the Framingham Study. *Am J Cardiol*. **38**: 46–51.
4 Kauffman SA (1993) *Origins of Order: self-organisation and selection in evolution.* Oxford University Press, New York.
5 Joint British Societies Coronary Risk Prediction Charts (1998) *British National Formulary*. Modified from: *Heart*. **80**: S1–S29.
6 Muir J, Fuller A, Lancaster T (1999) Applying the Sheffield tables to data from general practice. *Br J Gen Pract*. **49**: 217–18.
7 Dawkins R (1997) *Climbing Mount Improbable*. Penguin Books, London, pp. 89–93.
8 Eigen M, Winkler-Oswatitsch R (1996) *Steps Towards Life: a perspective on evolution*. Oxford University Press, Oxford.
9 Ridley M (1996) *Evolution* (2e). Blackwell Science, Cambridge, MA, pp. 215–20.
10 Holland JH (1995) *Hidden Order: how adaptation builds complexity*. Perseus Books, Cambridge, MA, pp. 69–76.
11 Anderson KM, Wilson PWF, Odell PM *et al.* (1991) An updated coronary risk profile. A statement for health professionals. *Circulation*. **83**(1): 356–62.
12 Dybowski R, Weller P, Chand R *et al.* (1996) Prediction of outcome in critically ill patients using artificial neural network synthesised by genetic algorithm. *Lancet*. **347**: 1146–50.
13 Holt TA, Ohno-Machado L (2003) A nationwide adaptive prediction tool for coronary heart disease prevention. *Br J Gen Pract*. **53**: 866–70.
14 National Service Frameworks (2000) *Coronary Heart Disease*. Chapter 2: Preventing coronary heart disease in high-risk patients. Department of Health, London.
15 Lapuerta P, Azen SP, LaBree L (1995) Use of neural networks in predicting the risk of coronary artery disease. *Computers and Biomedical Research*. **28**: 38–52.
16 Voss R, Cullen P, Schulte H *et al.* (2002) Prediction of risk of coronary events in middle-aged men in the Prospective Cardiovascular Münster Study (PROCAM) using neural networks. *International Journal of Epidemiology*. **31**: 1253–62.
17 Cross SS, Harrison RF, Lee Kennedy R (1995) Introduction to neural networks. *Lancet*. **346**: 1075–9.
18 SIGN (1999) *Lipids and the Primary Prevention of Coronary Heart Disease*. Scottish Intercollegiate Guidelines Network: Publication 40, Annex 9.

Conclusion

Tim Holt

There are many ironies in the history of complexity and chaos. A well known account describes how Edward Lorenz's 1963 paper on weather prediction[1] spent ten years in relative obscurity following its publication in the *Journal of the Atmospheric Sciences* before its much wider importance was recognised in the 1970s. With no disrespect to the journal, this example illustrates the regrettable fact that many of us are unlikely to find time to read material too far removed from our main subject areas. Much of what is written on non-linear dynamics (even that listed in major medical databases such as Medline) is published in journals that are outside the usual reading lists of practising clinicians. Some of this work is simply too technical for most of us to understand, but even the more accessible publications are unlikely to be actually encountered. Glass and Kaplan[2] have suggested the term 'dynamicist' as a possible new medical speciality (along with neurolog*ists*, cardiol-og*ists*, and the other *'ists'* of modern medical practice), and also the development of interdisciplinary groups to bridge this gap. The Complexity in Primary Care Group (www.complexityprimarycare.org), to which a number of this book's authors belong, explores the extension of these concepts into all areas of medicine – clinical care, organisational theory, public health, research methodology and others, to bring what is known closer to those practising and delivering healthcare.

My own interest in this subject originated as a teenager when my grandfather, a physicist and authority on light and visual perception, explained to me his research into the small eye movements on which we all depend to see the world in front of us. One of his books, *Eye Movements and Visual Perception*,[3] described the work he did to establish that when these movements are eradicated experimentally, visual perception fails. The conclusion intrigued me: an example of function that is utterly dependent on dynamical behaviour. This certainly questions the classical 'camera' model of the eye as a passive recipient of inflowing information from the outside world, and once again makes a case for movement and dynamism as healthy features of normal physiology.

But are these small eye movements random, or are they in fact as has been suggested,[4] an example of undiscovered chaos in physiology? My grandfather's book, published in 1973, describes in some detail what was known at the time, including a section on the movements' dynamics, without mentioning the term *chaos*, a term that I suspect would be important in a similar treatment of the subject today. So perhaps he himself might have benefited from Lorenz's insights of the decade before, had they been more widely circulated. This may be an indication of a change in perspective (and not just terminology) during the past 30 years, during which chaotic processes have been found to be commonplace in physiology. I don't know that this would be of any more than theoretical interest in the study of eye movements, but I hope we have demonstrated through this book that such a distinction might have very definite practical implications in certain clinical areas such as mental health, cardiology and diabetes, where an awareness of the underlying dynamical patterns provides a more adequate understanding of health and disease, as well as (at least in theory) an insight into the potential for, and limitations to, prediction, planning and the control of excessive variation.

Another major theme of this book has been to highlight the importance of *interactions* in the understanding of disease mechanisms and the provision of healthcare. Interactions are the feature of complex systems that generate creativity and emergent effects, but which preclude reductionist analysis and limit predictability. We have discussed interactions between the determinants of blood glucose, between risk factors, disease triggers, input variables in pattern recognition algorithms, sources of knowledge in decision making and between the members of a multidisciplinary healthcare team. Complexity is more about interactions than it is about anything. Complex behaviour arises even in simple systems provided interactions are non-linear. Indeed, it is this insight that stimulates the quest for simple rules underlying complex patterns.

Finally, in addition to dynamical patterns and interactions, the third major focus of this book has been the potential for *distributed pattern recognition* and its implications for the consultation, for decision making, multidisciplinary teamwork and for the integration of clinical databases in the twenty-first century.

Some of the concepts we have covered, as we saw in Part One, are difficult, and require a revision of some basic assumptions. But the increasing tendency towards specialisation requires us to unify our efforts through adequate communication and the sharing of knowledge not just within medicine, but between healthcare and the wider context. The study of complexity has penetrated a wide variety of scientific disciplines, in which the same basic principles have been seen to have relevance and applicability.[5] One of the objectives of this book has been to bring these theoretical insights to attention among clinicians, and apply them where appropriate to practical issues in everyday clinical practice.

References

1 Lorenz E (1963) Deterministic non-periodic flow. *Journal of the Atmospheric Sciences.* **20**: 130–41.
2 Glass L, Kaplan D (1993) Time series analysis of complex dynamics in physiology and medicine. *Medical Progress through Technology.* **19**(3): 115–28.
3 Ditchburn RW (1973) *Eye Movements and Visual Perception.* Oxford University Press, Oxford.
4 Rossler OE, Rossler R (1994) Chaos in physiology. *Integrative Physiological and Behavioural Science.* **29**(3): 328–33.
5 Gleick J (1987) *Chaos: making a new science.* Viking, New York.

Index